CURING YOGA

100+ HEALING YOGA SEQUENCES TO
ALLEVIATE OVER 50 AILMENTS

AVENTURAS DE VIAJE

Illustrated by
OKIANG LUHUNG

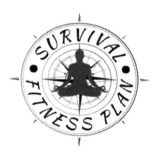

WARNINGS AND DISCLAIMERS

CONTENTS

SEQUENCES

HOW TO USE THIS BOOK

Besides the chapters on breathing and Yoga Nidra, this book is split into two main sections.

Poses

This section contains instructions on how to do all the poses mentioned in the sequences. They are in alphabetical order for easy reference.

Sequences

In the second section, you will find all the yoga sequences for curing your ailments. Each sequence has images and a list of poses that make up the sequence. The listed poses correlate to the images, with the first pose starting at the top left and the last finishing at the bottom right.

BREATHING

There are a few different types of breathing methods in yoga, but we only use two basic ones for all the routines in this book.

Three-Part Breath

This is the breath you will use most often when practicing yoga. Use it while doing the sequences in this book. When first learning it, you will probably want to do it from a sitting or lying position.

Breathe in long and deep through your nose. First, feel the breath enter your lower belly, then your lower chest/rib cage, and finally your lower throat/the top of your sternum. Feel the clear, positive energies of love and happiness come up from your toes to you head.

When you're ready, exhale fully through your nose, feeling the breath leave in the opposite order from the one it came in—first from your sternum, then your chest, and finally your belly. Release all tension and negative energies out of your body, from your head to your toes.

Continue to breathe in and out like this, smoothly and continuously.

When you first start to practice this type of breathing, it may help to put your hands on each of the three areas—your belly, chest, and sternum—as you do it. You can also try just breathing into each area on its own.

Alternate-Nostril Breathing

Alternate-nostril breathing is a quick and easy way to calm your nervous system and raise your happiness. It also helps clear congestion.

Sit tall and comfortably.

Curl the middle and index fingers of your right hand down into your palm.

Press your right ring finger on your left nostril to close it and breathe in to the count of four.

Now use your thumb to close off your right nostril so both your nostrils are closed. Count to four.

Release your ring finger and breathe out through your left nostril to the count of four.

Repeat this same sequence, but now breathe in through your right nostril.

Continue this alternation for three to five minutes.

YOGA NIDRA

Yoga Nidra is a form of guided meditation which has many health benefits. You can guide yourself, but the easiest way to do it is to listen to a Yoga Nidra practice and do what the instructor says.

For best results, find a place that isn't too hot or too cold, where your body can be comfortable and you can practice undisturbed. Put on some soothing background music if you want.

It is best not to do Yoga Nidra in bed, because you will be more likely to fall asleep. A yoga mat on the floor is ideal.

Yoga Nidra is a conscious practice.

Lie in Corpse Pose

Corpse pose, a.k.a. Shavasana, is a yoga pose used at the end of almost every yoga practice. Going straight from your yoga practice to Yoga Nidra is ideal and is (in my opinion) most likely the intention of the ones who created it.

Yoga Nidra can also be done from a seated position if lying down is inappropriate.

Close your eyes.

Corpse pose is explained in detail in the Poses section of this book.

Notice Your Breath

Notice your breathing. Feel your lungs filling with air, and your stomach expanding, and then deflating. Imagine a light around your body expanding and contracting as you breathe in and out. Feel the energy coursing through your body.

Use Your Senses

Notice each of your senses individually.

What sounds do you hear? Near, far, inside, outside.

What smells can you smell? Take small sniffs, like a dog does.

Taste the air.

Feel your body supported on the floor. Which parts of your body are touching?

What can you see with your eyes closed? Does the light make shapes in your eyelids?

Repeat Your Mantra

Your mantra is a short sentence stating your intentions. It's kind of like an affirmation. It may be an overall statement of health, relaxation, etc., or may be a visualization of something you want to achieve. One I use often is "My entire being is completely relaxed and at one with the universe." Whatever yours is, repeat it mentally three times. Try to feel how it would feel if the visualization was realized.

Scan Your Body

This is where you consciously relax each part of your body.

Mentally go through your body. Bring your attention to and relax each part. You can be very detailed about this, or just do large areas; it depends on how long you want to spend. I start from the top of my head and work my way down. Sometimes I even do my internal organs.

After you have relaxed smaller body parts, relax them as a whole. For example, after you've relaxed your shoulder, upper arm, bicep, elbow, forearm, hand, and fingers, relax your whole arm. At the end, relax your whole body as one.

Awaken the Body

The last step is to slowly deepen your breath and start to move your fingers and toes, then your hands and feet.

In your own time, stretch out your body out however feels right. Open your eyes when you're ready. When you are done stretching, gently hug your knees (wind-relieving pose). Fall to your right side and then gently sit up. Take a moment to reflect on the practice, and then go about your day.

POSES

Although all the poses used in this book are considered basic ones, you may find some of them challenging when you're first starting.

Adjust them to your comfort level and work your way up. Hold each pose to the point where you can feel a good stretch, but not pain.

You will probably notice your breath shorten if you try to force your body too much. When this happens, just back off a little and refocus on your breathing. If you do find yourself in a painful position, back out of it slowly to avoid injury.

ACCOMPLISHED POSE

Avoid this if you have a hip and/or knee injury.

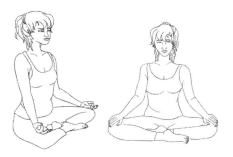

Sit with your buttocks on the floor, legs crossed.

Have both heels close to your midline by putting one foot near your inner thigh and the other one near your ankle.

Rest your hands in your lap or on your knees. Your palms can face up, down, or in a mudra.

Lengthen your spine by stretching the crown of your head towards the sky as you press your hips down.

Push your chest forward and drop your shoulders. Relax your whole face and belly.

BALANCING TABLE

Avoid this if you have an arm, back, knee, and/or shoulder injury.

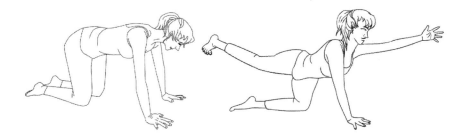

Place your hands and knees on the floor, with your palms directly underneath your shoulders and fingers facing forward. Your knees are shoulder-width apart and your feet are directly behind them. Have your back flat.

As you inhale, lift your right leg so it's parallel to the ground, with your toes pointing behind you.

Raise your left arm so it's also parallel to the ground, with your fingers pointing in front of you.

When you're ready, exhale as you bring first your arm and then your knee back into your starting position.

BOUND ANGLE

Avoid this if you have a hip and/or knee injury.

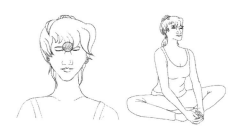

Start in a seated position with your legs extended straight out in front of you.

Bend your legs to bring the bottoms of your feet together. Your knees should bend outwards. Hold onto your toes by lacing your fingers around them.

As you inhale, stretch the crown of your head up towards the sky while pushing your hips down. Push your chest forward and relax your shoulders down.

Close your eyes and look to your third eye (behind the middle of your forehead). As you exhale, push your knees to the ground and gently pull your torso forward. Ensure you're keeping your chest open and your back flat.

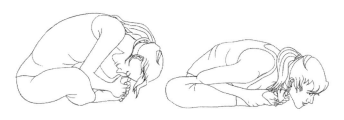

For a deeper stretch, pull your forehead or chest towards your feet. When you're ready, return to staff pose.

BRIDGE POSE

Avoid this if you have a back, knee, and/or shoulder injury.

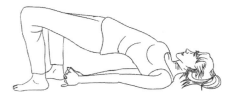

Lie down on your back and bend your knees up so that your feet are flat on the floor, hip-width apart.

Place your arms on the ground, straight but relaxed, palms down and with your fingertips just touching your heels.

As you inhale, push your feet into the ground and lift your hips up so that your spine rolls off the floor. Keep your knees hip-width apart.

Interlace your fingers underneath your back and lift your chest by pressing your arms and shoulders down. Use your buttocks, legs, and perineum muscles to lift your hips higher.

When you're ready, exhale and slowly roll your spine back to the ground.

CAT TILT

Avoid this if you have a back injury.

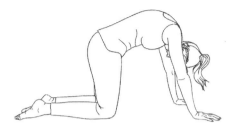

Place your hands and knees on the floor, with your palms directly underneath your shoulders and fingers facing forward. Your knees are shoulder-width apart and your feet are directly behind them. Have your back flat.

As you exhale, let your head and shoulders drop down and round your spine towards the sky.

You can inhale into dog tilt and exhale into cat tilt a couple of times before settling back into your starting position.

CATERPILLAR POSE

Avoid this if you have a back, elbow, neck, shoulder, and/or wrist injury.

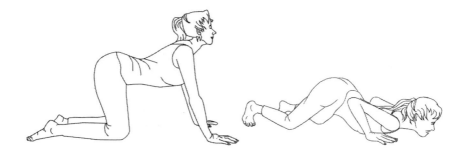

Place your hands and knees on the floor, with your palms directly underneath your shoulders and fingers facing forward. Your knees are shoulder-width apart and your feet are directly behind them.

As you inhale, arch your spine by letting your belly drop down and reaching your tailbone towards the ceiling.

Lower your chest and chin to the ground as you exhale. Your chest should be between your palms.

Push your chest to the ground as you raise your tailbone to the sky. Keep your elbows close to your sides.

You can inhale into dog tilt and exhale into the eight-limbed pose any number of times.

CORPSE POSE

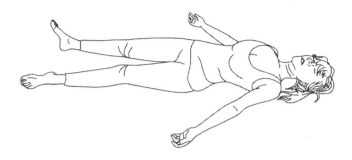

Lie flat on your back on the floor. You can place a pillow under your head if you want.

Keep your head straight; don't let it fall to the side.

Draw your shoulder blades down and open your chest towards your chin.

Have your arms at a comfortable distance from your body, with your palms facing up. Completely relax your arms and fingers.

Lift and extend your buttocks to your heels so that your whole sacrum rests on the floor.

Keep your abdomen soft and relaxed.

Slowly stretch your legs out straight, one at the time. Allow them to roll out to the side from the hips to the feet. Check that your body is in a straight line and you are resting evenly on the left and right sides.

Once you're comfortable, stay perfectly still and quiet and be aware of your body relaxing deeper into the floor. Allow your eyes to rest completely so they sink deeper towards the back of the skull. Relax your whole face and body. Be aware of your breath, quiet and soft.

CHAIR POSE

Avoid this if you have a back, hip, knee, and/or shoulder injury.

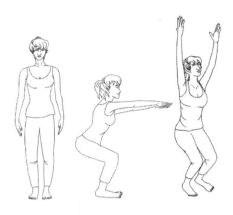

Stand with your feet parallel and either together or hip-width apart. Move your arms forward as you inhale so they are parallel to the ground.

Squat down at your knees as you breathe out. Have your knees pointing forward and shift your weight to your heels as you move your hips down and back. Ensure your hips don't sink below your knees. Pretend you're sitting on the edge of a chair.

Arch your spine by pressing your shoulders down and back. Relax your shoulders and stretch out through your fingertips. For more of a challenge, raise your arms to the sky and look up.

When ready, inhale as you straighten your legs and raise your arms to the sky, then exhale and lower your arms back to your starting position.

CHILD POSE

Avoid this if you have a knee injury.

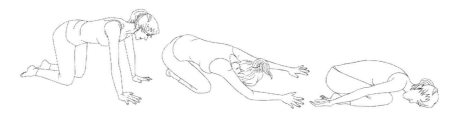

Place your hands and knees on the floor, with your palms directly underneath your shoulders and fingers facing forward. Your knees are shoulder-width apart and your feet are directly behind them. Have your back flat.

Lower your hips to your heels as you exhale and then place your forehead on the ground with your arms in front of you, palms facing down.

You can also put your arms down along the sides of your body with your palms facing up. Your knees can be together or slightly apart.

Press your belly against your thighs as you inhale.

When you're ready, place your palms under your shoulders and inhale as you come up to a seated position.

COBRA POSE

Avoid this if you have an arm, back, and/or shoulder injury, have had recent abdominal surgery, and/or are pregnant.

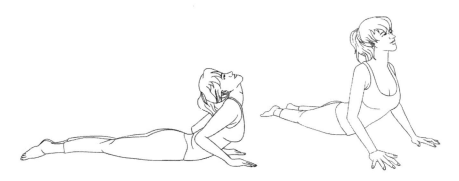

Lie on your stomach with your chin on the ground and your legs together.

Place your palms flat on the ground under your shoulders, elbows close to your sides.

Press your pubic bone into the ground and engage your buttocks, kneecaps, perineum, and thighs.

As you inhale, lift your head and chest off the ground without using your arms. Keep your neck and spine aligned. Now press down into your palms to lift yourself higher. Push your chest forward as you relax your shoulders back and down.

When you're ready, lower your chest and head back to the ground as you exhale.

CRAB POSE

Avoid this if you have an arm, back, hip, knee, and/or shoulder injury.

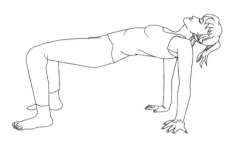

Start in a seated position with your legs extended straight out in front of you.

Place your hands behind your hips with your fingers facing forward. If you have wrist pain, you can make fists instead. Bend your knees up so that your feet are flat on the floor, hip-width apart, with your knees and toes pointing forward.

As you inhale, lean back into your arms and engage your whole body to lift your hips towards the sky. Look straight up to the sky or carefully allow your head to drop back.

When you're ready, exhale as you lower your hips back to the ground.

CRESCENT MOON

Avoid this if you have a back, hip, and/or shoulder injury.

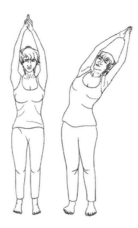

Stand with your feet parallel and either together or hip-width apart.

While inhaling, join your hands together above your head with your fingers interlaced and your index fingers pointing to the sky.

As you exhale, push your left hip out to the side and arch to your left. Keep your body strong and lengthened.

Inhale as you return to the position, with your fingers interlaced and your index fingers pointing to the sky. Repeat it on your other side.

CROCODILE POSE

Avoid this if you're pregnant.

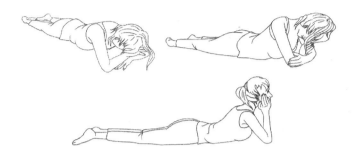

Lie on your stomach and cross your arms under your head, resting your forehead on your wrists. Alternatively, lift your torso up by crossing your arms with your elbows under your shoulders and then allowing your head to hang, or rest your chin in your palms with your elbows on the floor.

Allow your body to completely relax.

With each inhale, press your belly into the ground. With each exhale, relax your body more deeply.

DOG TILT

Avoid this if you have a back injury.

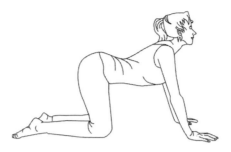

Place your hands and knees on the floor, with your palms directly underneath your shoulders and fingers facing forward. Your knees are shoulder-width apart and your feet are directly behind them. Have your back flat.

As you inhale, arch your spine by letting your belly drop down and reaching your tailbone towards the ceiling.

Press your palms into the ground as you spread your fingers wide apart. Drop your shoulders and look up to the sky, as high as you can without straining.

DOLPHIN POSE

Avoid this if you have an arm, back, and/or shoulder injury, glaucoma, and/or unmediated high blood pressure.

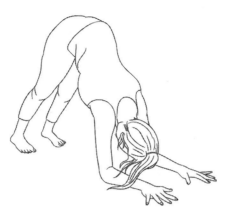

Place your hands and knees on the floor, with your palms directly underneath your shoulders and fingers facing forward. Your knees are shoulder-width apart and your feet are directly behind them. Have your back flat.

Get on the balls of your feet, lower your forearms to the ground, and lift your hips to the sky.

Ensure your palms and feet are shoulder-width apart, with your middle fingers and toes facing forwards. Spread your fingers as wide as you can.

Press into the floor with your hands and feet as you push your hips up and back. Ensure you keep your spine strong and lengthen it through your tailbone. Feel the stretch in the back of your legs. Keep your back straight. You can bend the backs of your knees a little if you need to.

Let your head hang and rest your forehead on the floor.

One-Legged Dolphin

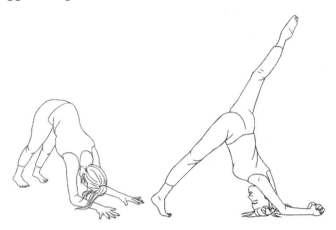

Starting from dolphin pose, lace your fingers together and raise one leg to the sky.

Stretch out through both your feet. That is, one into the ground and the other towards the sky.

DOWNWARD DOG

Avoid this if you have an arm, back, hip, and/or shoulder injury, and/or unmediated high blood pressure.

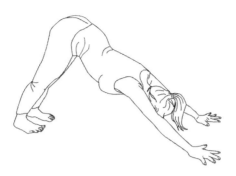

Place your hands and knees on the floor, with your palms directly underneath your shoulders and fingers facing forward. Your knees are shoulder-width apart and your feet are directly behind them. Have your back flat.

As you inhale, tuck in your toes so you are on the balls of your feet. Keep your palms shoulder width apart and spread your fingers apart, with your middle fingers facing forward.

Press into your hands and lift your hips towards the sky.

Push your hips up and back. Your chest should move towards your thighs. Keep your arms straight, but don't lock your elbows.

Keep your spine straight as you lift up through your tailbone.

Stretch the backs of your legs by pressing your heels to the floor. Keep your back flat. Your legs should be straight (knees not locked) or with a small bend at the knees.

Let your head dangle freely.

DOWNWARD-FACING FROG

Avoid this if you have a knee, hip, and/or leg injury.

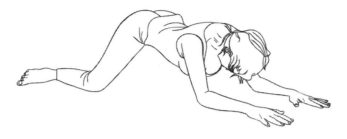

Kneel on the ground with your knees together and your feet hip-width apart. Sit with your bum on the ground and your heels on the outside of your hips.

Spread your knees as wide as you comfortably can and align your feet so that they are directly behind them—that is, with your right foot behind your right knee and your left foot behind your left knee.

Turn your feet outwards so your toes are facing away from your body.

Place your elbows, forearms, and palms flat on the floor.

Exhale as you push your hips back.

EXTENDED DOG

Avoid this if you have an arm, back, knee, and/or shoulder injury.

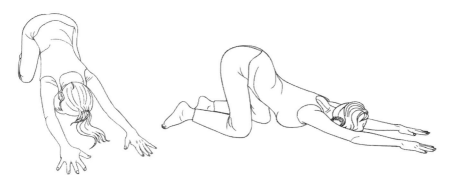

Place your hands and knees on the floor, with your palms directly underneath your shoulders and fingers facing forward. Your knees are shoulder-width apart and your feet are directly behind them. Have your back flat.

As you inhale, push your tailbone towards the sky then exhale and lower your forehead to the floor by sliding your hands forward. Ensure you keep your hips lifted over your knees.

Arch the middle of your back by allowing your chest to sink towards the floor.

Deepen the stretch by straightening your arms, lifting your elbows off the floor, and bringing your hips back. Try not to let your hands slide while you do this.

Place your chin on the ground to stretch your neck.

When you're ready, inhale and return to your starting position.

EXTENDED SIDE ANGLE

Avoid this if you have a hip, knee, neck, and/or shoulder injury.

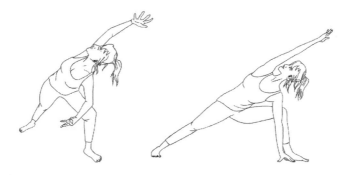

Adopt a lunge position with your left foot forward and your left elbow resting on your left knee.

As you inhale, raise your right arm to the sky, and then as you exhale, lengthen it over your ear, so that the right side of your body is a straight line. You could also bring your left hand to the ground on either side of your foot.

Allow your hips to sink to the ground as you reach through the fingers of your right hand. Ensure your left knee is directly over your left ankle.

FISH POSE

Avoid this if you have an arm, back, neck, and/or shoulder injury.

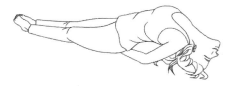

Lie on your back with your legs slightly apart and your arms along the side of your body.

Slide your hands under the tops of your thighs. Your elbows should be slightly bent, facing out from the sides of your torso.

Roll onto the crown of your head by pressing your arms into the ground as you arch your spine and lift your chest.

Place little to no weight on your head and neck. Let the rest of your body do the work.

FIVE-POINTED STAR

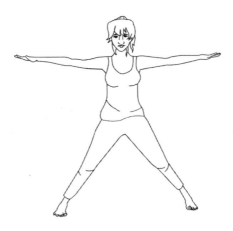

Stand with your feet parallel and either together or hip-width apart.

Lift your arms out to the sides and set your feet wide apart so that they're under your wrists and facing forward.

Press your weight down into your feet and set your legs solidly onto the floor.

Relax your shoulders, moving them down and back as you push your chest forward.

As you inhale, extend your body up through your crown, down through your feet, and out through your hands.

GATE POSE

Avoid this if you have a hip, knee, and/or shoulder injury.

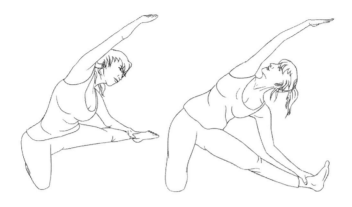

Kneel down, with your knees hip-width apart.

Point your left leg straight out to your left, foot flat on the ground and toes pointing to the left. Rest your left palm on your left leg.

As you inhale, raise your right arm to the sky.

As you exhale, drop your right arm over your ear and slide your left arm to your toes. Keep your arms straight.

Lengthen your body by pressing out through your right hip, pushing into your foot and knee, and reaching out through your fingers and the crown of your head. Keep your chest open and either look straight ahead or up to the sky.

When you're ready, inhale, bringing your right arm and knee back to a kneeling position.

HALF-BOW

Avoid this if you have an arm, hip, leg, and/or neck injury, have had recent abdominal surgery, and/or are pregnant.

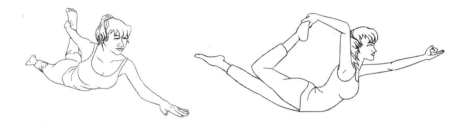

Lie on your stomach with your chin on the floor and your hands over your head, palms facing down. Have your legs either together or just a little apart.

Bend your left knee and grab onto your ankle or heel with your right hand.

As you inhale, lift your left leg, chest, and head off the ground. Ensure your neck is in line with your spine and look to your third eye.

Your left arm can either be on the ground in front of you or lifted in the air, parallel to the ground.

When you're ready, exhale as you let your body sink back into the ground.

HALF-CAMEL

Avoid this if you have a back, knee, neck, and/or shoulder injury, have had recent abdominal surgery, and/or have a hernia.

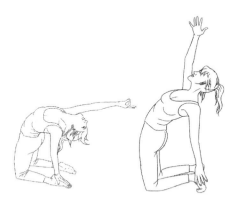

Get on your knees with your palms on your sacrum, fingers pointing to the ground. Ensure your knees are hip-width apart. Your feet can either be flat or with your toes tucked.

As you inhale, lengthen your spine by pushing the crown of your head to the sky while pressing your knees down.

Press your hips forward and bend backwards as you exhale.

Use your arms to support your weight and very carefully grab your left heel or foot with your left hand. If it's too challenging to grab your foot, you can keep your hand on your sacrum.

As you inhale, reach your right hand behind you, and if you're comfortable doing so, gently drop your head back. If that's too challenging, you can point your hand to the sky.

When you're ready, place both hands back on your sacrum and inhale as you come back to a kneeling position. Bring your head and neck up last.

HALF-CIRCLE

Avoid this if you have an arm, hip, knee, and/or shoulder injury, and/or if you have a hernia.

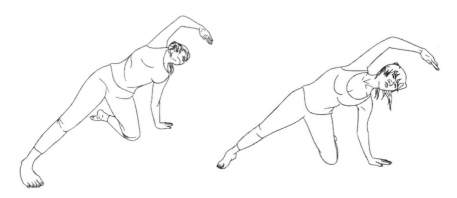

Kneel down with your knees hip-width apart.

Point your right leg straight out to the side, foot flat on the floor, and toes facing forwards.

Gently lower your left hand to the ground so it's directly under your left shoulder.

As you inhale, bring your right hand over your head, palm facing the ground.

Arch your spine as you push your hips forward and let your head drop back.

Reach out through the fingers of your left hand as you push your left foot into the ground. The left side of your body should make a half-circle shape.

When you're ready, bring your arms parallel to the floor as you inhale, and then, as you exhale, bring your hands to your hips and step back into a kneeling position.

HALF-FORWARD FOLD

Avoid this if you have a back, hip, and/or shoulder injury.

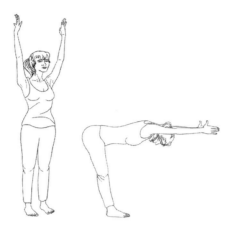

Stand with your feet parallel and either together or hip-width apart. Raise your hands above your head with your palms facing each other.

As you exhale, bend forward at your hips until your torso is parallel with the ground. Keep a flat back as you do this.

Lengthen your hips, shifting them back and your crown and fingers forward. Keep your legs strong.

HALF-LOCUST

Avoid this if you have a back and/or leg injury, have had recent abdominal surgery, and/or are pregnant.

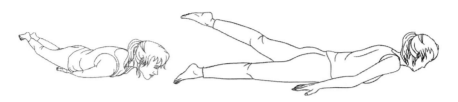

Start by lying on your belly, legs together and arms relaxed along the side of your body, palms facing the ground. Rest your chin on the floor.

Bring your hands under your body so that they're under your thighs, with your forearms on the inside of your hipbones. It may help to rock your body from side to side as you inch your arms in. If this is too uncomfortable, you can leave your arms alongside your body.

As you inhale, lengthen your legs and toes, stretching them back. Engage your pelvic area and your upper legs as you press your arms into the ground and lift them up to the sky. If that's too challenging, just lift one leg at a time.

When you're ready, exhale as you gently relax back to the ground. Turn your head to one side and bring your arms out from under your body.

HALF PRAYER-TWIST

Avoid this if you have a back, hip, knee, and/or shoulder injury.

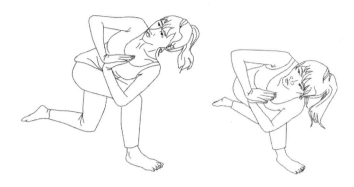

Adopt a low lunge position with your right foot forward and your left lower leg flat on the ground. Place your palms on the floor, one on each side of your front foot.

As you inhale, bring your torso up and place your hands together in a prayer position.

Place your left elbow to the outside of your right knee and use your arms to press your left shoulder up and back. Feel it twist your upper back.

Ensure your palms remain in the center of your chest with your fingers pointing towards your throat.

You can either look straight ahead or up towards the sky.

When you're ready, exhale as you bring your palms back to the floor, one on each side of your left foot.

HALF-PYRAMID

Avoid this if you have a knee and/or leg injury.

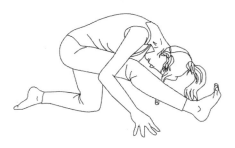

Adopt a low lunge position with your right foot forward and your left lower leg flat on the ground.

While exhaling, straighten your right leg as you press your hips back towards your left heel.

Round your spine and lift your toes to the sky as you push your forehead into your right knee. Walk your hands back towards you to support your torso. Relax your elbows, face, neck, and shoulders.

When you're ready, inhale and bend your right knee back over your ankle, and then exhale and bring your right knee back next to your left one.

HALF SHOULDER-STAND

Avoid this if you have a back, neck, and/or shoulder injury, are menstruating or pregnant, and/or have unmediated high blood pressure.

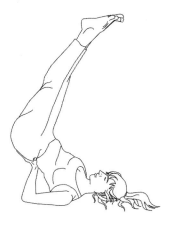

Lie on your back and place your arms along the sides of your body, palms facing down.

Bend your knees and rock back to bring them to your forehead. As you do this, place your hands under your hips and cup them for support.

Lift your legs up to straighten them over your head.

You should have very little weight on your head and neck. Support yourself with your arms.

Find the spot where you're balanced and then relax your legs.

When you're ready, bend your knees to your head and gently roll your spine back onto the floor.

HALF-SUPINE HERO

Avoid this if you have a knee injury.

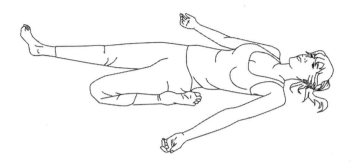

Kneel on the ground with your knees together and your feet hip-width apart. Sit with your bum on the ground and your heels on the outside of your hips. Extend your right leg in front of you.

Carefully walk your hands behind you and lower yourself to the floor: first onto your elbows, then the crown of your head, and eventually onto the back of your neck. Only go as low as you feel comfortable going.

Once you're on your back, rest your hands at the sides of your body.

When you're ready, grab your left foot with your left hand and apply pressure to slowly bring yourself back up to a seated position.

HALF WIND-RELIEVING POSE

Avoid this if you have a hernia and/or have had recent abdominal surgery.

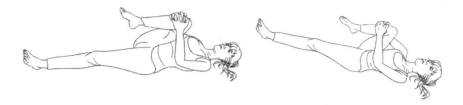

Lie on your back.

As you inhale, bring your right knee to your chest and hold it there by placing your fingers around it, just below the kneecap.

Tuck your chin to your chest, with your head on the floor, and gently pull your right knee into your chest. Avoid your ribcage when doing this.

Keep your elbows close to your body, and push your shoulders and the back of your neck into the floor. Relax your lower body.

As you inhale, press your belly into your thigh.

When you're ready, release everything to the floor as you exhale.

HALF-UPRIGHT SEATED ANGLE

Avoid this if you have a hip, knee, and/or shoulder injury.

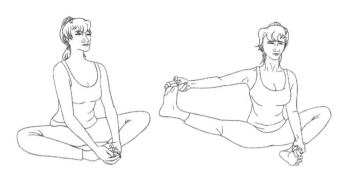

Start in a seated position with your legs bent to bring the bottoms of your feet together. Grab your big toes with the middle and index finger of each hand.

As you inhale, lift your right foot off the floor and put it straight to your right. Press out through your heel.

Keep your torso vertical by pulling gently on your left foot.

Push your chest forward and relax your shoulders, shifting them down and back.

When you're ready, exhale as you bend your right knee and bring your feet back to your starting position.

HERO POSE

Avoid this if you have a knee injury.

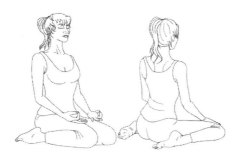

Kneel on the ground with your knees together and your feet hip-width apart. Sit with your bum on the ground and your heels on the outside of your hips. If this is too difficult, you can sit on your heels.

Place your hands on your knees. Your palms can face up or down.

Lengthen your torso by reaching the crown of your head to the sky.

Push your lower legs into the ground, drop your shoulders, and press your chest forward.

Relax your belly, face, jaw, and tongue.

Hero pose is an excellent pose for rest and/or meditation.

HIGH PLANK

Avoid this if you have an arm, back, and/or shoulder injury.

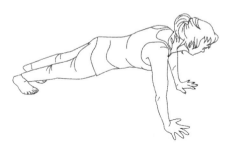

Go into the "up" position of a pushup. Spread your fingers wide apart, middle finger facing forward, and press your hands into the ground.

Keep your arms straight, but not locked at the elbow. Tense your bum so that your body forms a straight line.

Push back onto your heels as you lengthen through the crown of your head.

JOYFUL BABY

Avoid this if you have a leg, neck, and/or shoulder injury.

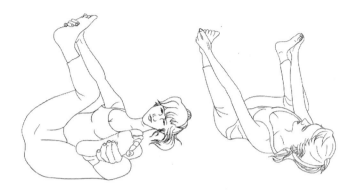

Lie flat on your back on the floor.

As you inhale, bring your knees to your chest.

Weave your arms through the inside of your knees and hold onto the pinkie-toe sides of your feet with your hands.

Keep your head on the ground and tuck your chin to your chest.

Push your heels up to the sky as you pull back with your arms. At the same time, press the back of your neck, shoulders, sacrum, and tailbone to the floor.

Open your legs wider for a deeper hip stretch.

When you're ready, exhale and slowly roll your spine back to the ground until you're lying flat again.

KNEE-DOWN TWIST

Avoid this if you have a back, hip, and/or knee injury.

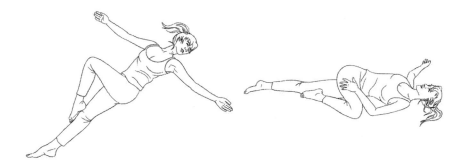

Lie on your back and extend your arms out to your sides at right angles to your torso, palms facing down.

Bend your left knee and place your left foot over your right knee.

As you exhale, twist your lower body to the right and allow your left knee to drop over your right leg.

Look towards the fingers of your left hand or straight up. Relax into the posture, allowing gravity to do the work.

For more of a stretch, you can put your right hand on your left knee to add more weight. You don't need to push down on it.

When you're ready, inhale as you untwist to a straight back and exhale as you lower your leg down to the floor.

LION POSE

Avoid this if you have a face, knee, neck, and/or tongue injury.

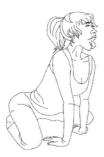

Kneel on the ground with your knees together and your feet hip-width apart. Sit with your bum on the ground and your heels on the outside of your hips.

Bring your feet together and spread your knees as wide as you comfortably can.

Sit on your heels.

Inhale and lengthen your spine by stretching the crown of your head towards the sky.

Bring your palms to the floor in between your knees, with your fingers facing your body.

Arch your spine, stick your tongue out, and exhale ferociously via your mouth.

Repeat this a few times.

LOW WARRIOR

Avoid this if you have an ankle, arm, hip, and/or shoulder injury.

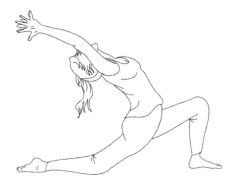

Place your hands and knees on the floor, with your palms directly underneath your shoulders and fingers facing forward. Your knees are shoulder-width apart and your feet are directly behind them. Have your back flat.

Step your right foot forward, placing it in between your hands. Your knee should be directly over your ankle.

Ensure your left knee and left and right feet are firmly on the ground, and then place your hands on your right knee.

Straighten your arms and bring your torso back. Do not lock your elbows.

Relax your shoulders and stick your chest out by bringing your shoulder blades towards each other.

As you inhale, raise your arms over your head with your palms facing each other and arch your back as you look up to the sky. If this is difficult, then you can keep your hands on your bent knee.

When you're ready, exhale as you bring your palms back to the floor on either side of your right foot.

MOUNTAIN POSE

Avoid this if you have a shoulder injury.

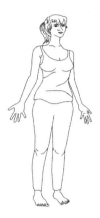

Stand with your feet parallel and either together or hip-width apart.

Spread your toes wide and balance your weight evenly and centrally over each foot.

Pull up your kneecaps and tense your thighs. Keep your legs straight, but do not lock your knees. Ensure your hips are directly over your ankles.

As you inhale, lengthen your spine so that the crown of your head goes straight up towards the sky.

When you exhale, drop your shoulders and stretch your fingertips towards the ground, whilst still extending your head upwards. At the same time, gently push your chest straight ahead.

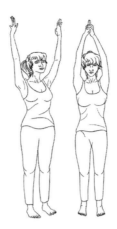

While continuing to stretch your fingertips, inhale and bring your arms up above your head to reach for the sky, palms facing each other.

As you exhale, relax your shoulders, but continue to stretch your crown and fingers towards the sky. An alternative position is to interlace your fingers with your index fingers pointing up.

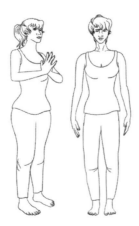

When you're ready, exhale and bring your palms together in front of your chest in a prayer position. Take a breath, and allow your hands to drop to your sides on the exhale.

ONE-HANDED TIGER

Avoid this if you have a back, hip, knee, and/or shoulder injury.

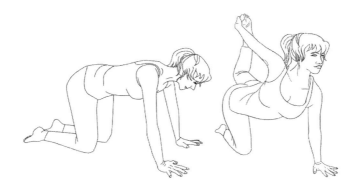

Place your hands and knees on the floor, with your palms directly underneath your shoulders and fingers facing forward. Your knees are shoulder-width apart and your feet are directly behind them. Have your back flat.

As you exhale, keeping your knee bent and gently arching your spine, extend your left foot to the sky.

Put your weight over your left hand and use your right hand to hold onto the inside of your left foot or ankle.

Keep both arms straight and look straight ahead. Gently lift your left leg higher.

When you're ready, exhale as you return to your starting position.

PIGEON POSE

Avoid this if you have a back, hip, and/or knee injury.

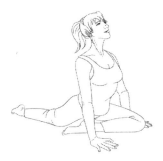

Place your hands and knees on the floor, with your palms directly underneath your shoulders and fingers facing forward. Your knees are shoulder-width apart and your feet are directly behind them. Have your back flat.

Slide your left knee between your hands and allow your left foot to slide to over to the right. Shift your right leg back and lower your hips towards the ground.

As you inhale, press into your hands and lengthen your spine by pressing the crown of your head to the sky. Drop your hips into the ground as you exhale. Push out through your chest and roll your shoulders back and down. To increase the stretch, slide your left foot further away from your hips.

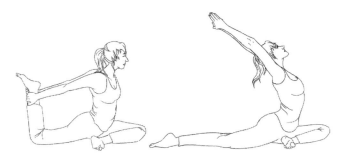

Variations of the Pigeon Pose

Extended Pigeon Pose

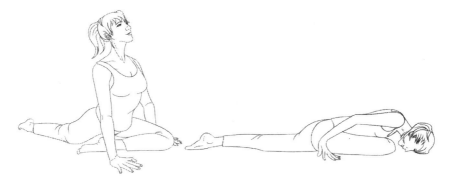

Slowly lower your head and chest to the ground by walking your hands forward.

If you can't put your head on the ground support, it with your hands, placing them between it and the floor.

When you're ready, walk your hands back up until you're back in pigeon pose.

PRAYER SQUAT

Avoid this if you have a hip and/or knee injury.

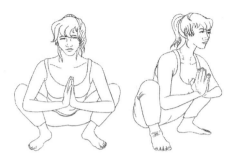

Stand with your feet parallel and hip-width apart. Put your palms together in front of your chest in a prayer position. Spread your legs about hip-width apart and squat down all the way.

Shift your feet a little further apart if needed, until your torso isn't resting on your thighs. If you're able, have your feet flat on the ground.

Lengthen your spine by sinking your hips into the ground as you stretch the crown of your head to the sky. Push your chest forwards and roll your shoulders down and back.

If you can do so without losing balance, close your eyes and look to your third eye.

PYRAMID POSE

Avoid this if you have a back, hip, and/or shoulder injury.

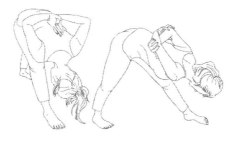

Start in a lunge position with your left foot forward.

Step back with your right foot to straighten both of your legs. Make sure your rear foot is flat, with your toes facing forwards.

Push your forehead towards your left knee as you press the back of your knees and your heels to your rear.

If you're able, bring your hands behind your back either in a prayer position or holding onto your elbows.

RABBIT POSE

Avoid this if you have a knee, neck, shoulder, and/or spine injury.

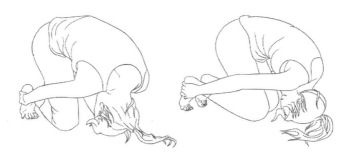

Place your hands and knees on the floor, with your palms directly underneath your shoulders and fingers facing forward. Your knees are shoulder-width apart and your feet are directly behind them. Have your back flat.

Lower your hips to your heels as you exhale and then place your forehead on the ground with your arms in front of you, palms facing down.

Grab onto your heels and place the top of your head on the ground. Pull your forehead to your knees.

As you inhale, lift your hips to the sky.

Roll onto the crown of your head and try to get your forehead as close to your knees as you can.

SEATED ANGLE

Avoid this if you have an arm, hip, knee, and/or shoulder injury.

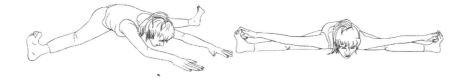

Start in a seated position with your legs extended straight out in front of you.

As you inhale, spread your legs out as wide as comfortable.

Ensure your knees and toes are pointing up and reach through your fingers up to the sky.

Exhale as you lower your palms to the floor.

Deepen the stretch by walking your hands forward. Stay focused on keeping your spine long. You could also hold your big toes and use them to help pull your torso down.

When you're ready, inhale and slowly walk your hands in as you roll back your spine until you finish with a straight back.

SEATED FORWARD BEND

Avoid this if you have an ankle, arm, hip, and/or shoulder injury.

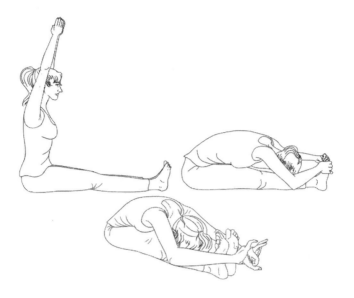

Start in a seated position with your legs extended straight out in front of you. Inhale and raise your arms up to the sky, with your palms facing each other. Lengthen your torso through your fingers and the crown of your head.

As you exhale, bend at the hips, lowering your upper body to your legs. Grab your ankles, feet, or toes.

Push out through your heels as you pull your toes back towards you.

You can use your arms to pull yourself closer to your legs. If you have more flexibility, reach your hands in front of your feet. If you're having difficulties, bend your knees enough so that you can reach your feet and place your head on your knees.

When you're ready, slowly roll up your spine back into the seated position.

SEATED HEAD-TO-KNEE POSE

Avoid this if you have a back and/or knee injury.

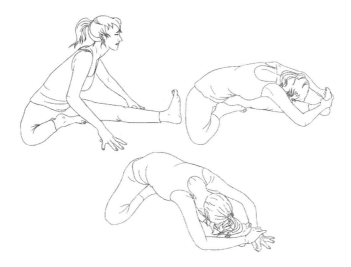

Start in a seated position with your left leg out in front of you. Put the bottom of your right foot up against your left thigh and have your hips square.

As you inhale, raise your arms up and lengthen your spine by stretching up through the crown of your head and your fingertips. Continue to lengthen as you exhale and bend forward at your hips. Lace your fingers around your right foot, bending your knee if you need to.

Press your head down into your knee and push your left heel away from you in an effort to straighten your leg. Pull your toes back towards you. Relax your upper body. Only use your arms as much as needed to keep your head in contact with your knee. To increase the stretch, reach your hands past your foot and grab your wrist.

When you're ready, inhale with your arms back over your head and then exhale as you bring them to the ground.

SEATED SPINAL TWIST

Avoid this if you have a back, hip, and/or shoulder injury.

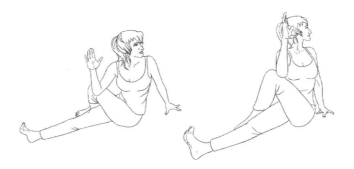

Start in a seated position with your legs extended straight out in front of you. Cross your left leg over your right and place your left foot flat on the floor near your right knee.

Wrap your right arm around your left knee and pull it into your chest. Lengthen your spine by pushing up through the crown of your head and down through your waist.

As you inhale, raise your left hand up. Exhale as you place it on the ground behind you, fingers facing back. Keep your back straight by pressing your arm into it.

Look over your left shoulder as you place your right elbow on the outside of your left knee.

Inhale and lengthen your spine. As you exhale, use your arms to increase the twist. Relax your shoulders and push your chest out to open it.

When you're ready, inhale as you lift your left hand up and untwist your body to face forward.

SIDE SEATED ANGLE

Avoid if you have a hip, leg, and/or lower back injury.

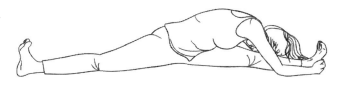

Start in a seated position with your legs spread your legs out as wide as comfortable.

Turn to face your right foot by twisting at your waist.

Walk your hands towards your right foot as you exhale. Try to reach your forehead to your knee and hold your right ankle or foot if you are able.

Relax your shoulders and neck and then increase the stretch by pressing your heel out while pulling your toes back towards yourself.

When you're ready, return to center with your back straight and then do the same thing on your left side.

STAFF POSE

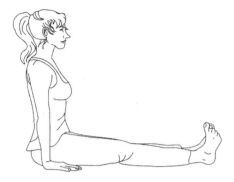

Start in a seated position with your legs extended straight out in front of you. Place your hands beside your hips with your fingers pointed forward.

Lengthen your spine by pressing your hip bones down while pushing the crown of your head towards the sky. Use your arms for support as you push your chest forward and lower your shoulders.

Pull your toes towards your head as you push your heels away from you.

STANDING BACKBEND

Avoid this if you have a back, hip, and/or neck injury.

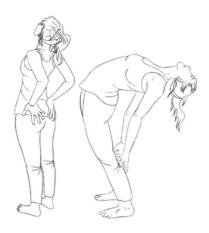

Stand with your feet parallel and hip-width apart.

As you breathe in, place the palms of your hands on your lower back (sacrum) with your fingers pointing to the ground.

Squeeze your buttocks and thighs tightly together, pull up your kneecaps, and press into your feet.

Exhale and press your hips forward as you arch your back.

You can either look straight ahead or allow your head to drop all the way back.

Increase the stretch by walking your hands down the back of your legs.

When you're ready, slowly come back to a standing position with your hands by your sides.

STANDING FORWARD FOLD

Avoid this if you have a back, hip, leg, and/or shoulder injury.

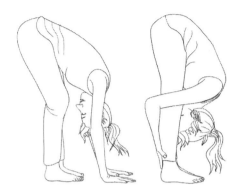

Stand with your feet parallel and either together or hip-width apart.

Exhale and bring your head to your knees, with your palms flat on the floor.

Stretch your spine by pulling your head down while pushing your hips up. Bend your knees if you need to, but aim to be able to do it with straight legs. Press your belly into your thighs when inhaling.

For a deeper stretch, hold the back of your calves and pull your head closer to your legs.

STANDING YOGA SEAL

Avoid this if you have a back, leg, neck, and/or shoulder injury, and/or unmediated high blood pressure.

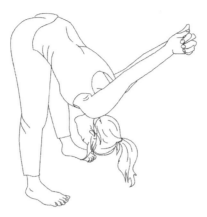

From a standing position, lift your arms out to the sides and set your feet wide apart so that they're under your wrists and facing forward.

Inhale as you interlace your fingers behind you.

Draw your shoulders back to expand your chest and look up to the sky.

As you exhale, keep your legs and arms straight and bend forward at your hips. Reach your arms up and forward and allow your head to hang.

Keep your weight distributed evenly over your feet. To make the pose harder, bring your feet closer together.

When you're ready, inhale as you come back up and exhale as you release your arms.

SUPINE BOUND ANGLE

Avoid this if you have a hip and/or shoulder injury.

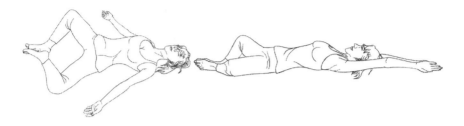

Lie flat on your back on the floor. Bend your legs to bring the bottoms of your feet together.

Your knees should face out just like in bound angle, but lying down. Allow your knees to drop to the ground.

You can rest your hands on your thighs to "encourage" them, but don't push down.

As you inhale, slide your arms on the ground over your head until your palms are together. Cross your thumbs.

When you're ready, exhale as you return to a lying position.

TABLE POSE

Avoid this if you have a knee and/or wrist injury.

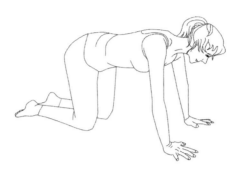

As you inhale, place your hands and knees on the floor, with your palms directly underneath your shoulders and fingers facing forward.

Ensure your knees are shoulder-width apart and your feet are directly behind them, with the tops of your feet and toes on the floor.

Look at the ground between your hands and press down into your palms.

Have your back flat and exhale while lengthening your spine by pressing the crown of your head forward and your tailbone back.

THREADING THE NEEDLE

Avoid this if you have a knee, neck, and/or shoulder injury.

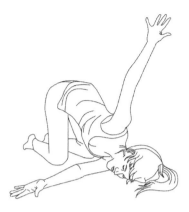

Place your hands and knees on the floor, with your palms directly underneath your shoulders and fingers facing forward. Your knees are shoulder-width apart and your feet are directly behind them. Have your back flat.

As you exhale, slide your right hand between your left knee and left hand until your right shoulder and the side of your head are resting on the floor.

Inhale and reach towards the sky with your left hand. Find where you get the deepest stretch and stay there, reaching out with your fingers.

When you're ready, exhale as you bring your hand back to the floor and then inhale to readopt your starting position.

Repeat on your left side.

TREE POSE

Avoid this if you have a hip and/or knee injury.

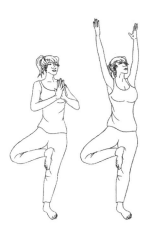

Stand with your feet parallel and either together or hip-width apart and then shift all your weight over your left leg.

Bend your right knee so that your right heel rests on your left leg.

Slide your right foot up your left leg as high as you can without losing your balance. Point your toes to the ground.

Bring your hands together in prayer position.

Press your chest forward and your left foot into the ground.

If you're able, inhale and bring your hands above your head, palms facing each other. Reach up through your fingers.

When you're ready, exhale as you return to a standing position.

TRIANGLE POSE
Avoid this if you have a back, hip, and/or shoulder injury.

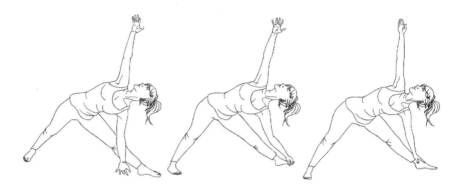

From a standing position, lift your arms out to the sides and set your feet wide apart so that they're under your wrists and facing forward.

Point your left toes to your left and turn the toes of your right foot slightly inwards.

As you inhale, push your hip to the right and slide your arms to the left so they are parallel to the floor.

Rotate your arms as you exhale, resting your left hand against your left leg and raising your right arm up, palms facing forward.

Make a straight line with your arms and stretch out with your fingertips. Press your feet into the ground. Your left hand can be on the ground, grabbing your toes, or on your ankle.

When you're ready, inhale as you return to your starting position.

UPWARD BOAT

Avoid this if you have an abdomen, hip, knee, and/or shoulder injury.

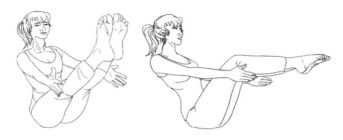

Sit down on your bum with your knees bent and feet flat on the floor.

Put your legs together and place your hands behind your hips, with your elbows bent away from you and your fingers pointing forwards.

Lift your heels off the ground a little by leaning back. Open your chest by drawing your shoulder blades together. Slowly straighten your legs and lift them as high as you're comfortable doing.

Extend your arms forward, palms facing the floor and parallel to the ground.

Continue to lift your chest with the same amount of effort as you use to lift your legs. If this is too challenging, keep your knees bent and/or your hands on the floor.

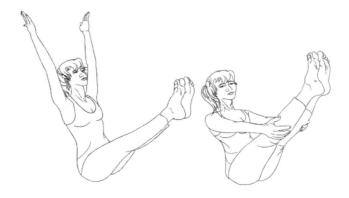

You can also reach both your hands above your head or hold onto the back of your knees.

When you're ready, exhale as you bend your knees and then lower your feet back to the ground.

UPWARD DOG

Avoid if you have an arm, back, hip, and/or shoulder injury, have had recent abdominal surgery, and/or are pregnant.

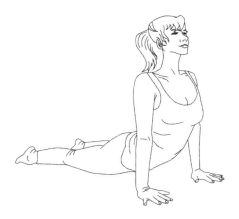

Place your hands and knees on the floor, with your palms directly underneath your shoulders and fingers facing forward. Your knees are shoulder-width apart and your feet are directly behind them. Have your back flat.

Drop your hips forward towards the ground as you press your palms down into the floor.

Press your chest forward as you drop your shoulders down and back.

Push the crown of your head towards the ceiling.

As you inhale, press the tops of your feet into the ground to lift your legs off the floor. Only the tops of your feet and your hands should touch the ground. Press all of your toenails firmly into the floor.

UPWARD FORWARD FOLD

Avoid this if you have an arm, back, and/or shoulder injury.

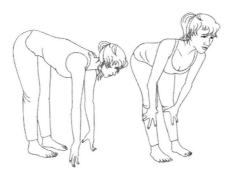

Allow your hands to dangle down to the ground. Place your hands on the floor if they reach.

As you inhale, arch your back and look to the sky.

Extend your nose forward, push your sternum to the floor, and lengthen your tailbone behind you.

If you're having difficulties, bring your hands to your knees.

WARRIOR ONE

Avoid this if you have a back, hip, knee, and/or shoulder injury.

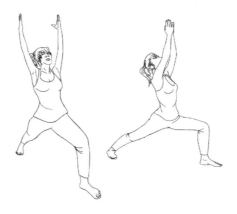

From a standing position, lift your arms out to the sides and set your feet wide apart so that they're under your wrists and facing forward.

Bend your left knee and turn to face your left.

Turn your right foot 45 degrees and keep your heel on the floor. The heel of your front foot and the arch of your rear foot are lined up.

Ensure your left knee is directly over your ankle, with your hips and shoulders square and facing forwards.

As you inhale, raise your arms above your head, with your palms facing each other. Keep your shoulders relaxed and your chest lifted. Go deeper by bringing your palms together and carefully arching your back as you look to the sky.

Press into your feet and extend through your fingers and crown as you exhale.

When you're ready, exhale as you lower your hands down to the floor.

WARRIOR TWO

Avoid this if you have a hip, knee, and/or shoulder injury.

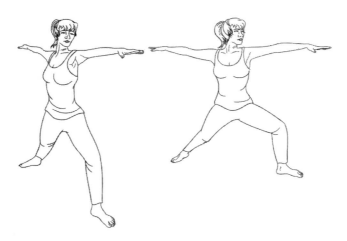

From a standing position, lift your arms out to the sides and set your feet wide apart so that they're under your wrists and facing forward.

Bend your left knee directly over your left ankle, turning your left foot so your toes face to your left.

Keep your right foot planted into the ground as you turn to look toward the fingers of your left hand.

Push your chest forward and relax your shoulders.

Lengthen your spine by stretching the crown of your head to the sky and sinking your hips to the ground.

WIDE-LEGGED FORWARD BEND

Avoid this if you have a back, hip, leg, and/or shoulder injury.

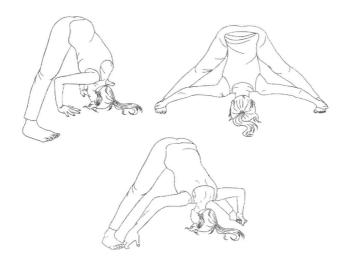

From a standing position, lift your arms out to the sides and set your feet wide apart so that they're under your wrists and facing forward.

Exhale and bend at your waist to bring your palms to the ground under your shoulders.

Keep your back straight.

Widen your legs if you need to in order to make your hands reach the floor.

Bend your elbows to your rear as you pull your forehead towards the ground.

Push your feet into the ground and raise your hips to the sky. You can also hold onto your feet or toes.

When you're ready, inhale and shift back up into your starting position.

WIND-RELIEVING POSE

Avoid this if you have a hernia and/or have had recent abdominal surgery.

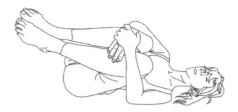

Lie flat on your back on the floor.

As you inhale, bring both knees up to your chest.

Hug your knees and hold onto the elbows, forearms, fingers, or wrists of your opposite arm (that is, hold your right arm with your left hand, and vice versa).

Keep your head on the floor while tucking your chin to your chest.

Pull your knees to your chest as you press the back of your neck, shoulders, sacrum, and tailbone to the floor. Relax your feet, hips, and legs.

Inhale deeply into your belly and press it against your thighs as you do so.

When you're ready, exhale and relax all your limbs to the ground so you are lying flat again.

SEQUENCES

How long each of these sequences takes is up to you. Stay in each pose for as long as you like.

While doing the sequences, use deep breathing techniques such as three-part breath. This is a very important part of yoga.

Unless otherwise stated, when doing a pose on one side, do it on the opposite side immediately afterwards as well.

If you don't know how to do a pose, you can learn how to do it in the first section of this book. Once you know all the poses in a sequence, aim to flow from one to the next regardless of the starting position for each individual pose.

Note: If you ever find yourself in a painful position, back out of it slowly to avoid injury.

SUN SALUTATION

This is a classic vinyasa yoga sequence to warm your body up at the start of a yoga session.

It is also a great sequence to do as a general yoga practice when you have no specific ailment to work on.

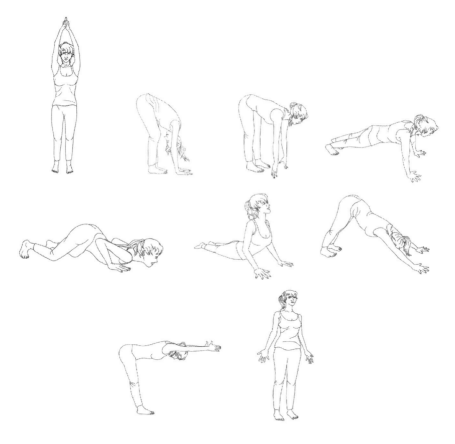

Mountain Pose - Standing Forward Fold - Upward Forward Fold - High Plank - Caterpillar Pose - Cobra Pose - Downward Dog - Half-Forward Fold - Mountain Pose

ACHES AND PAINS

This is a very general sequence to help with mild body aches and pains.

Be sure to breathe, move slowly, and pay attention to what your body is telling you.

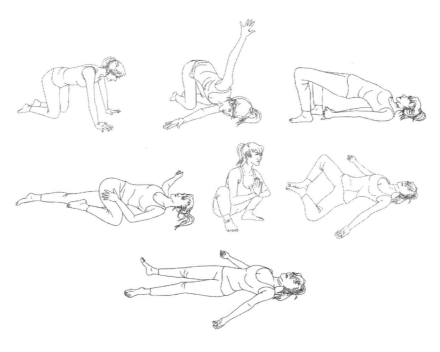

Table Pose - Threading the Needle - Bridge - Knee-Down Twist - Prayer Squat - Supine Bound Angle - Corpse Pose

ACNE

Try this routine daily and eat a healthy diet for best results.

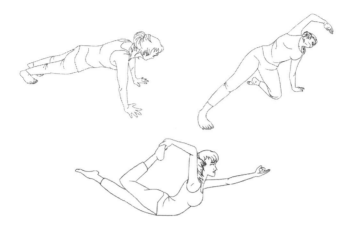

High Plank - Half-Circle - Half-Bow

ADD/ADHD

These quick routines are also good for anybody with a cluttered mind, such as you might have after an extra-hard day at work.

ADD/ADHD Sequence One

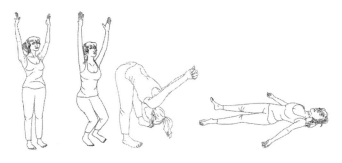

Mountain Pose - Chair Pose - Standing Yoga Seal - Corpse Pose

ADD/ADHD Sequence Two

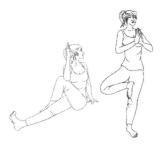

Seated Spinal Twist - Tree Pose

ALLERGIES

Do this routine twice daily when you experience allergy symptoms.

This sequence is also good to do at least three times a week for building up your general immunity. See the sequences for cold and flu, and immunity as well.

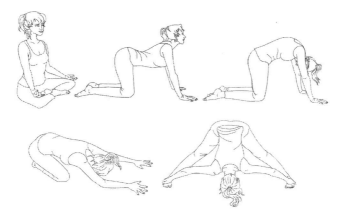

Accomplished Pose (with alternate nostril breathing) - Dog Tilt - Cat Tilt - Child Pose - Wide-Legged Forward Bend

ARTHRITIS

The following sequence is very general. You may wish to add poses depending on your problem area.

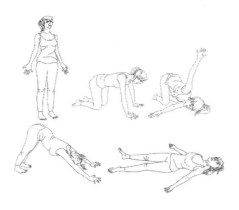

Mountain Pose - Table Pose - Threading the Needle - Downward Dog - Corpse Pose

ASTHMA

While doing this sequence, pay special attention to opening your chest. See the respiratory ailments sequence as well.

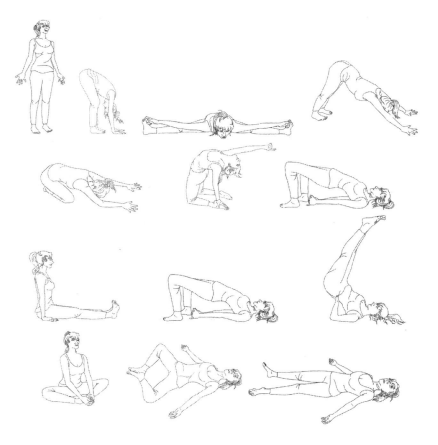

Mountain Pose - Standing Forward Fold - Seated Angle - Downward Dog - Child Pose - Half-Camel - Bridge Pose - Staff Pose - Bridge Pose - Half Shoulder-Stand - Bound Angle - Supine Bound Angle - Corpse Pose

BACKACHE

Be very careful when doing sequences for backache. Move slowly, never strain or hold your breath, and keep your neck and facial muscles relaxed.

Backache Sequence One

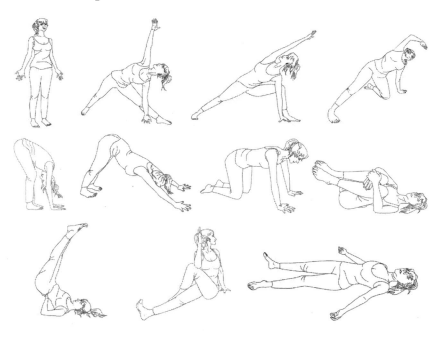

Mountain Pose - Triangle Pose - Extended Side Angle - Half-Circle - Standing Forward Fold - Downward Dog - Table Pose - Wind-Relieving Pose - Half Shoulder-Stand - Seated Spinal Twist - Corpse Pose

Backache Sequence Two

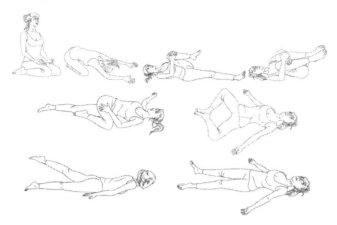

Hero Pose - Child Pose - Half Wind-Relieving Pose - Wind-Relieving Pose -
Knee-Down Twist - Supine Bound Angle - Half-Locust - Corpse Pose

Backache Sequence Three

This sequence is specifically helpful for the upper back and neck.

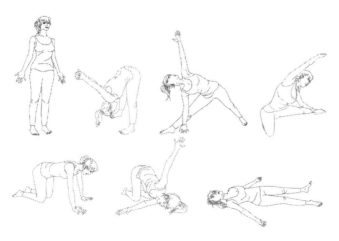

Mountain Pose - Standing Yoga Seal - Triangle Pose - Gate Pose - Table Pose
- Threading the Needle - Corpse Pose

BALANCE

This sequence improves balance in your mind and body.

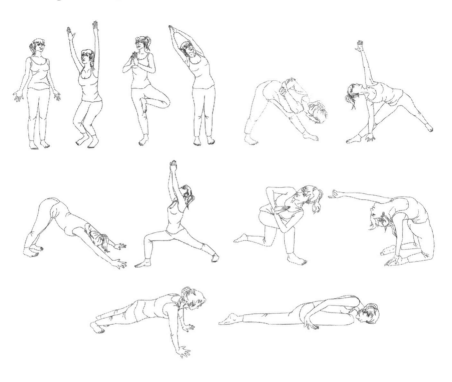

Mountain Pose - Chair Pose - Tree Pose - Crescent Moon - Pyramid Pose - Triangle Pose - Downward Dog - Warrior One - Half Prayer-Twist - Half-Camel - High Plank - Extended Pigeon Pose

BROKEN HEART

When you feel broken-hearted, do this sequence daily until you feel better.

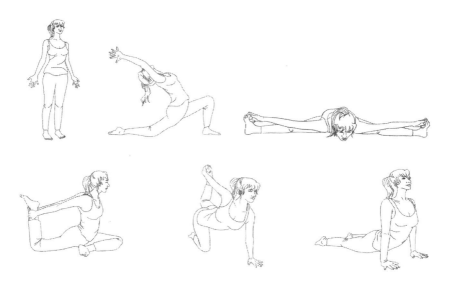

Mountain Pose - Low Warrior - Seated Angle - Pigeon Pose - One-Handed Tiger - Upward Dog - Bridge Pose

CHANGE

This sequence will help you adjust to times of change in all areas of life.

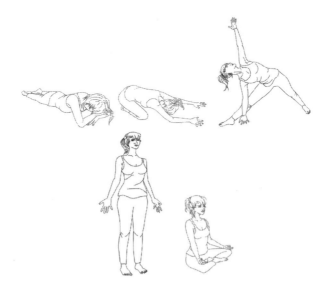

Crocodile Pose - Child Pose - Triangle Pose - Mountain Pose - Accomplished Pose (with meditation)

CIRCULATION

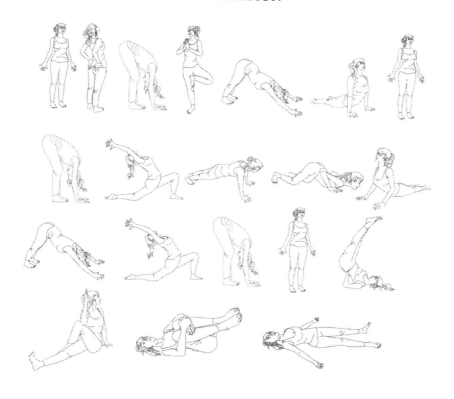

Mountain Pose - Standing Backbend - Standing Forward Fold - Tree Pose - Downward Dog - Upward Dog - Mountain Pose - Standing Forward Fold - Low Warrior (right side) - High Plank - Caterpillar Pose - Cobra Pose - Downward Dog - Low Warrior (left side) - Standing Forward Fold - Mountain Pose - Half Shoulder-Stand - Seated Spinal Twist - Wind-Relieving Pose - Corpse Pose

COLD AND FLU

Both of these sequences are useful for cure and prevention of colds, since they also strengthen your immune system in general. While doing them, pay special attention to opening your chest.

See the sequences for allergy and immunity as well.

Cold and Flu Sequence One

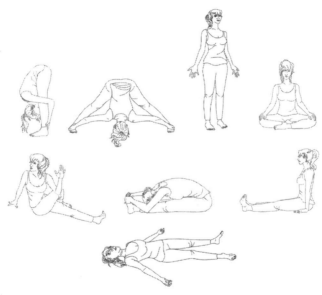

Standing Forward Fold - Wide-Legged Forward Bend - Mountain Pose - Accomplished Pose (with alternate nostril breathing) - Seated Spinal Twist - Seated Head-to-Knee Pose - Staff Pose - Corpse Pose

Cold and Flu Sequence Two

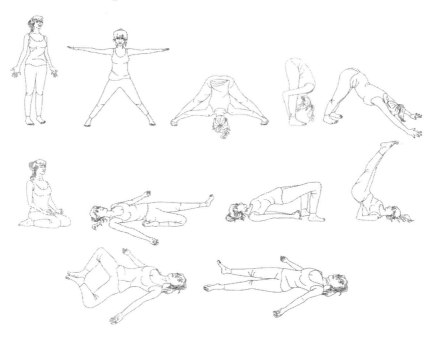

Mountain Pose - Five-Pointed Star - Wide-Legged Forward Bend - Standing Forward Fold - Downward Dog - Hero Pose - Half-Supine Hero - Bridge Pose - Half Shoulder-Stand - Supine Bound Angle - Corpse Pose

COMPLEXION

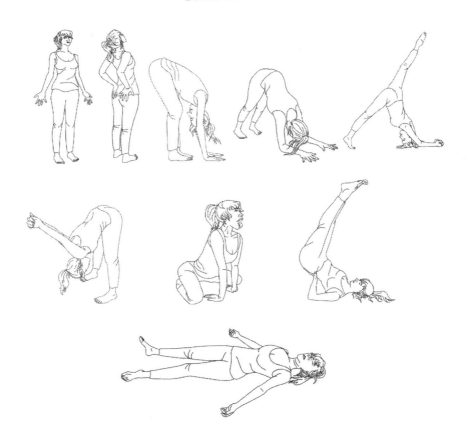

Mountain Pose - Standing Backbend - Standing Forward Fold - Dolphin Pose - One-Legged Dolphin - Standing Yoga Seal - Lion Pose - Half Shoulder-Stand - Corpse Pose

CRAVINGS

Whatever your craving or addiction (alcohol, cigarettes, drugs, sugar, etc.), this sequence can help.

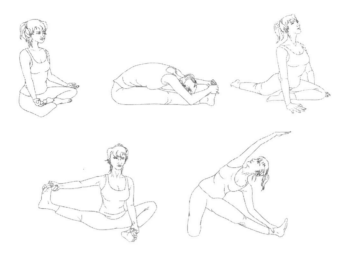

Accomplished Pose - Seated Forward Bend - Pigeon Pose - Half-Upright Seated Angle - Gate Pose

DEPRESSION

Any of these sequences can be used for long-term depression or even just a quick pick-me-up when you're feeling a little down.

Depression Sequence One

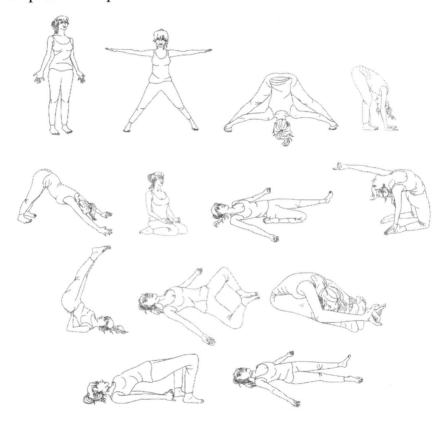

Mountain Pose - Five-Pointed Star - Wide-Legged Forward Bend - Standing Forward Fold - Downward Dog - Hero Pose - Half-Supine Hero - Half-Camel - Half Shoulder-Stand - Supine Bound Angle - Seated Forward Bend - Bridge Pose - Corpse Pose

Depression Sequence Two

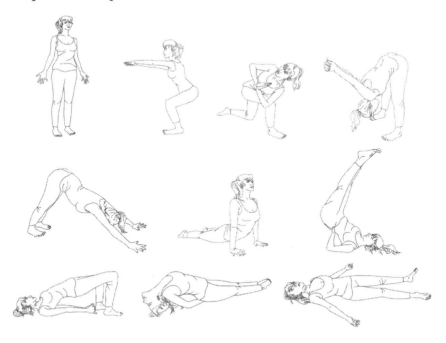

Mountain Pose - Chair Pose - Half-Prayer Twist - Standing Yoga Seal - Downward Dog - Upward Dog - Half Shoulder-Stand - Bridge Pose - Fish Pose - Corpse Pose

Depression Sequence Three

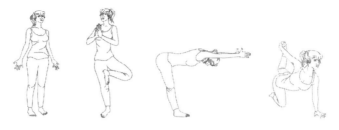

Mountain Pose - Tree Pose - Half Forward Fold - One-Handed Tiger

Depression Sequence Four

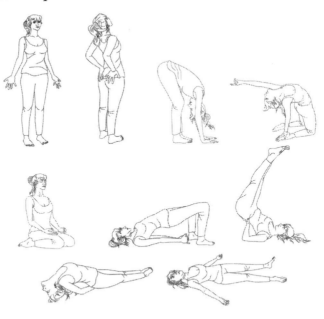

Mountain Pose - Standing Backbend - Standing Forward Fold - Half-Camel
- Hero Pose - Bridge Pose - Half Shoulder-Stand - Fish Pose - Corpse Pose

FIBROMYALGIA

When you're doing this sequence, it's especially important to pay attention to your breath. Concentrate on relaxing your muscles as well.

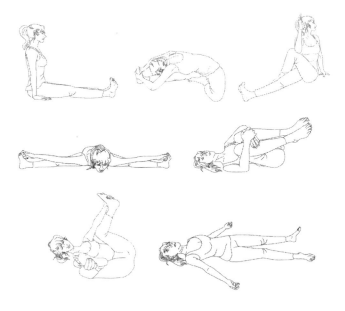

Staff Pose - Seated Head-to-Knee Pose - Seated Spinal Twist - Seated Angle - Wind-Relieving Pose - Joyful Baby - Corpse Pose

FOOT CRAMPS

To soothe a sudden spate of foot cramps, squat down and sit on your heels with your toes tucked.

If you have a bit more time, use the following sequence which also helps with prevention when done a few times a week.

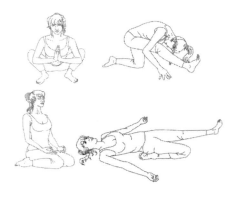

Prayer Squat (on balls of feet) - Half-Pyramid - Hero Pose - Half-Supine Hero

HANGOVER

Handstands aren't included in this book, as they're considered more than a basic pose, but they are great for headaches and hangovers, so do them if you can.

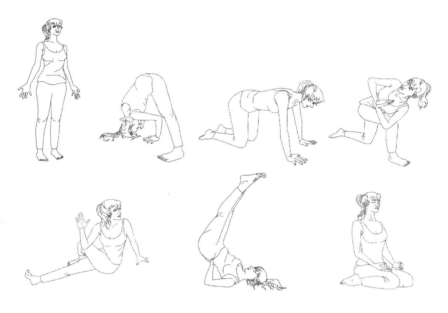

Mountain Pose - Wide-Legged Forward Bend - Table Pose - Half Prayer-Twist - Seated Spinal Twist - Half Shoulder-Stand - Hero Pose

HEADACHE AND MIGRAINE

The following sequences are good for everyday headaches, as well as for chronic migraines. They can also be done regularly to help keep migraines away for good.

When doing these sequences, focus on keeping your brain quiet and lengthening your neck.

Headache/Migraine Sequence One

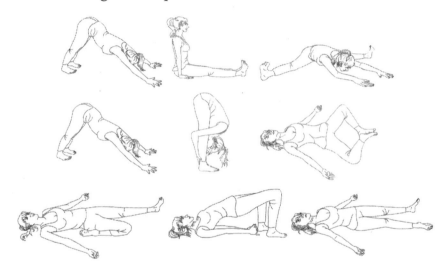

Downward Dog - Staff Pose - Seated Forward Bend - Downward Dog - Standing Forward Fold - Supine Bound Angle - Half-Supine Hero - Bridge Pose - Corpse Pose

Headache/Migraine Sequence Two

To do a temple massage, use your index fingers to press on your third eye, then trace two opposing lines to your temples with your fingers. Repeat this several times.

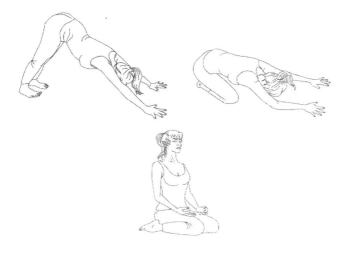

Downward Dog - Child Pose - Hero Pose (with temple massage)

HEART AND LUNGS

This sequence is not for any specific ailment, but will help to strengthen your heart and lungs in general.

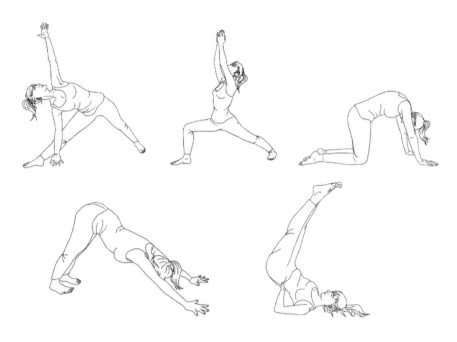

Triangle Pose - Warrior One - Cat Tilt - Downward Dog - Half Shoulder-Stand

HIGH BLOOD PRESSURE

If you have high blood pressure be sure to check with your physician before starting any new exercise regime, including yoga.

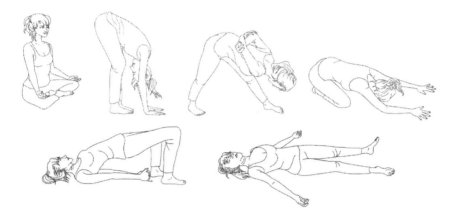

Accomplished Pose (with alternate nostril breathing) - Standing Forward Fold - Pyramid Pose - Child Pose - Bridge Pose - Corpse Pose

HIP DISCOMFORT

Hip Discomfort Sequence One

This sequence is specifically for stiff hips and can also be used to prevent arthritis of the hips.

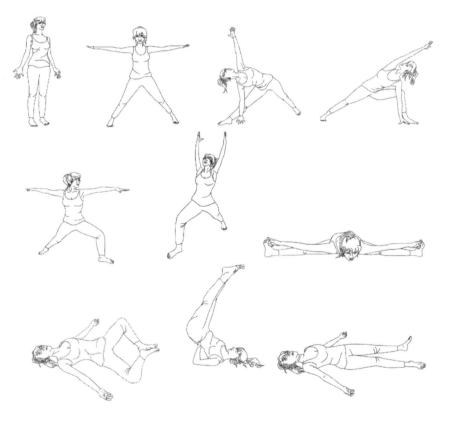

Mountain Pose - Five-Pointed Star - Triangle Pose -
Extended Side Angle - Warrior Two - Warrior One
Seated Angle - Supine Bound Angle - Half Shoulder-Stand - Corpse Pose

Hip Discomfort Sequence Two

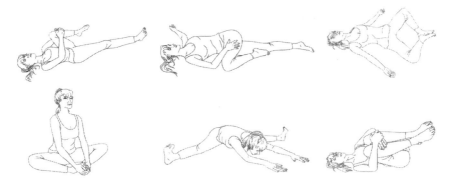

Half Wind-Relieving Pose - Knee-Down Twist - Supine Bound Angle -
Bound Angle - Seated Angle - Wind-Relieving Pose

IMMUNITY

See the sequences for allergies, cold, and flu as well.

Immunity Sequence One

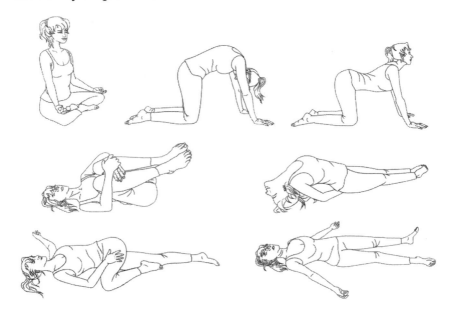

Accomplished Pose - Dog Tilt - Dog Tilt - Wind Relieving Pose - Fish Pose -
Knee Down Twist - Corpse Pose

Immunity Sequence Two

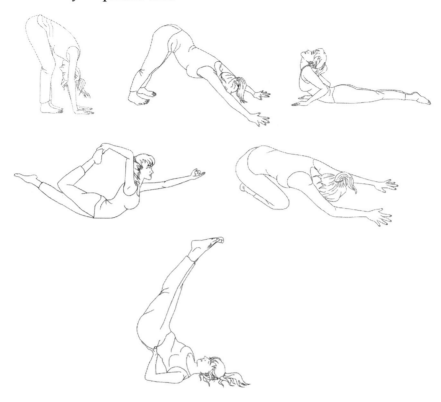

Standing Forward Fold - Downward Dog - Cobra Pose - Half-Bow - Child Pose - Half Shoulder-Stand

INDIGESTION

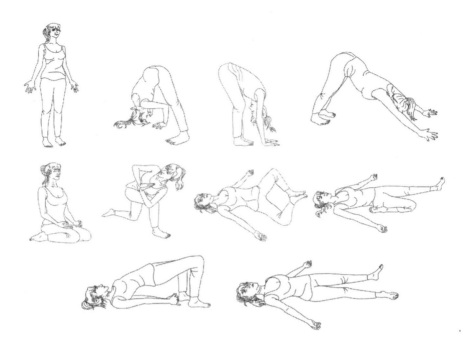

Mountain Pose - Wide-Legged Forward Bend - Standing Forward Fold - Downward Dog - Hero Pose - Half Prayer-Twist - Supine Bound Angle - Half-Supine Hero - Bridge Pose - Corpse Pose

INSOMNIA

Do these routines before going to bed.

Insomnia Sequence One

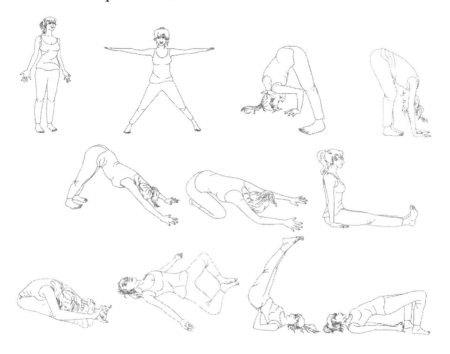

Mountain Pose - Five-Pointed Star - Wide-Legged Forward Bend - Standing Forward Fold - Downward Dog - Child Pose - Staff Pose - Seated Forward Bend - Supine Bound Angle - Half Shoulder-Stand - Bridge Pose

Insomnia Sequence Two

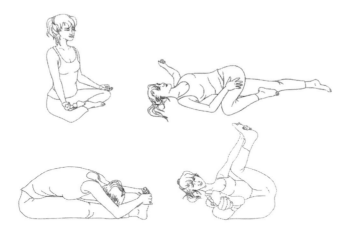

Accomplished Pose (with meditation) - Knee-Down Twist - Seated Forward Bend - Joyful Baby

KNEE PROBLEMS

When doing these sequences, keep your legs strong and engaged. This will create space in the knee joint and provide support. Be careful not to make any jerking movements.

Knee Problems Sequence One

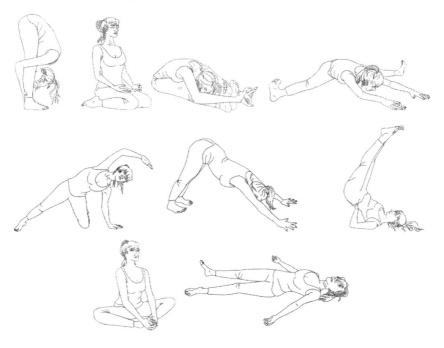

Standing Forward Fold - Hero Pose - Seated Forward Bend - Seated Angle - Half-Circle - Downward Dog - Half Shoulder-Stand - Bound Angle - Corpse Pose

Knee Problems Sequence Two

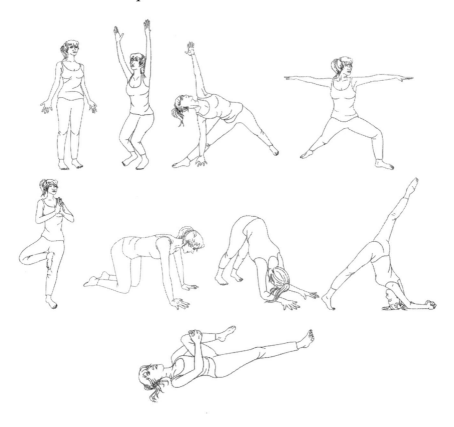

Mountain Pose - Chair Pose - Triangle Pose - Warrior Two - Tree Pose - Table Pose - Dolphin Pose - One-Legged Dolphin - Half Wind-Relieving Pose

LETHARGY

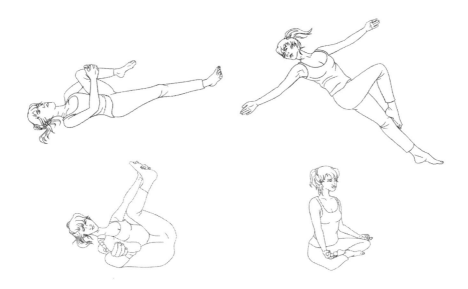

Half Wind-Relieving Pose - Knee-Down Twist - Joyful Baby - Accomplished Pose

LONG TRAVEL

You can use these routines anytime you have been sitting for a long time.

Long Travel Sequence One

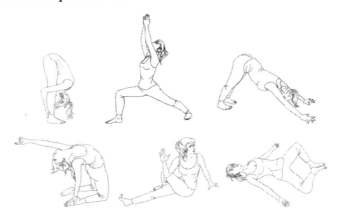

Standing Forward Fold - Warrior One - Downward Dog - Half-Camel - Seated Spinal Twist - Supine Bound Angle

Long Travel Sequence Two

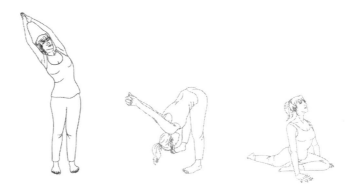

Crescent Moon - Standing Yoga Seal - Pigeon Pose

LOW SELF-ESTEEM

Low Self-Esteem Sequence One

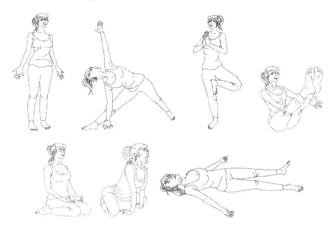

Mountain Pose - Triangle Pose - Tree Pose - Upward Boat - Hero Pose - Lion Pose - Corpse Pose (with Yoga Nidra)

Low Self-Esteem Sequence Two

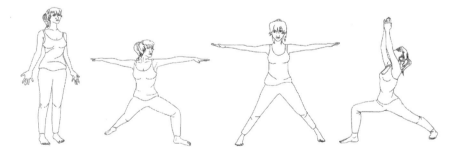

Mountain Pose - Warrior Two - Five-Pointed Star - Warrior One

Low Self-Esteem Sequence Three

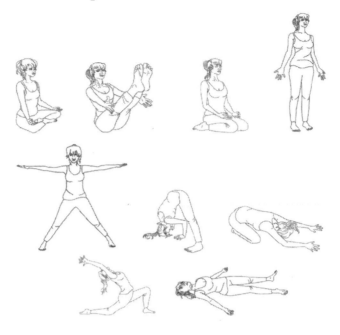

*Accomplished Pose (with meditation) - Upward Boat - Hero Pose -
Mountain Pose - Five-Pointed Star - Wide-Legged Forward Bend - Child
Pose - Low Warrior - Corpse Pose (with Yoga Nidra)*

Low Self-Esteem Sequence Two

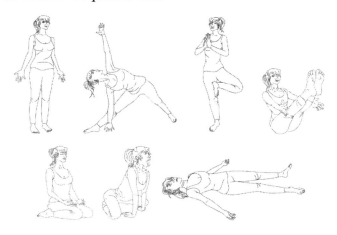

Mountain Pose - Triangle Pose - Tree Pose - Upward Boat - Hero Pose - Lion Pose - Corpse Pose (with Yoga Nidra)

Low Self-Esteem Sequence Three

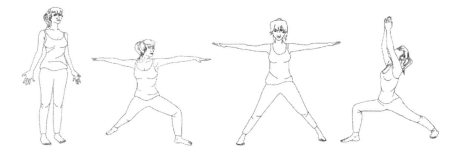

Mountain Pose - Warrior Two - Five-Pointed Star - Warrior One

MENOPAUSE AND HOT FLASHES

Menopause

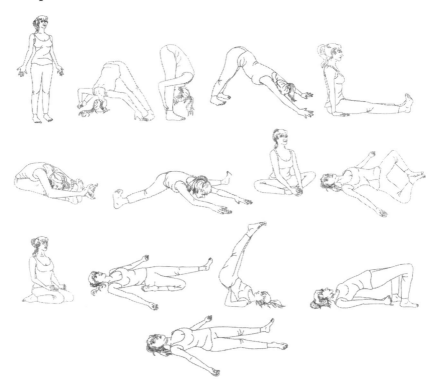

Mountain Pose - Wide-Legged Forward Bend - Standing Forward Fold - Downward Dog - Staff Pose - Seated Forward Bend - Seated Angle - Bound Angle - Supine Bound Angle - Hero Pose - Half-Supine Hero - Half Shoulder-Stand - Bridge Pose - Corpse Pose

Hot Flashes

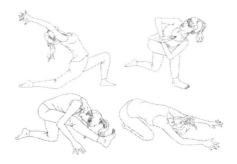

Low Warrior - Half Prayer-Twist - Half-Pyramid Pose - Child Pose

MENSTRUATION

The following sequences can relieve discomforts you may feel during menstruation, and if used regularly, they can have permanent effects.

Menstruation Sequence One

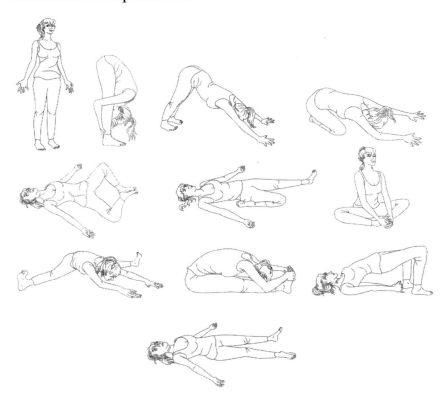

Mountain Pose - Standing Forward Fold - Downward Dog - Child Pose -
Supine Bound Angle - Half-Supine Hero Pose - Bound Angle - Seated Angle
- Seated Forward Bend - Bridge Pose - Corpse Pose

Menstruation Sequence Two

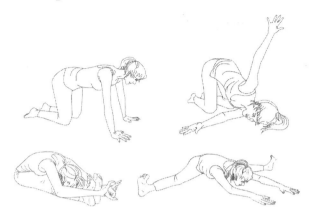

Table Pose - Threading the Needle - Seated Forward Bend - Seated Angle

Menstruation Sequence Three

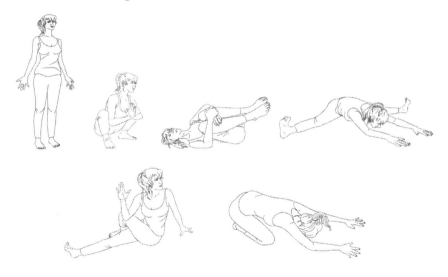

Mountain Pose - Prayer Squat - Wind-Relieving Pose - Seated Angle -
Seated Spinal Twist - Child Pose

POSTURE

In order to correct your posture, you need to do the following routine regularly. Concentrate on having an open chest with your shoulders down and back.

Posture Sequence One

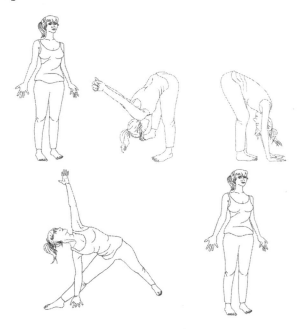

Mountain Pose - Standing Yoga Seal - Standing Forward Fold - Triangle Pose - Mountain Pose

Posture Sequence Two

This sequence focuses more on spinal alignment and flexibility.

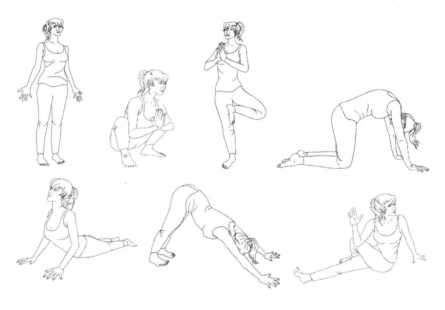

Mountain Pose - Prayer Squat - Tree Pose - Cat Tilt - Cobra Pose - Downward Dog - Seated Spinal Twist

PREGNANCY

Care must be taken when doing any physical activity during pregnancy, and it is no different for yoga.

Do not do twists, especially during your first trimester. It's also best to avoid inversions (headstands, handstands, etc.)

It is highly recommended to seek advice from a professional yoga instructor as well as your doctor to discover the best way to continue your yoga practice while you're pregnant. That said, these two gentle routines can be done in any phase of pregnancy.

Pregnancy Sequence One

Go for a walk after completing this routine.

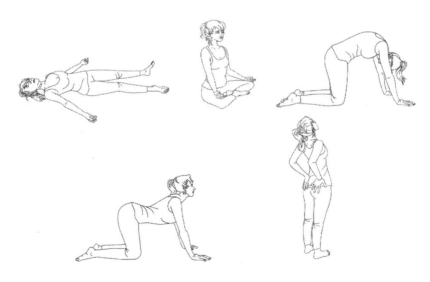

Corpse Pose (with meditation) - Accomplished Pose - Cat Tilt - Dog Tilt - Standing Backbend

Pregnancy Sequence Two

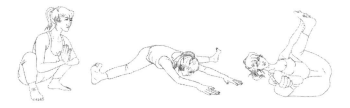

Prayer Squat - Seated Angle - Joyful Baby

PROCRASTINATION

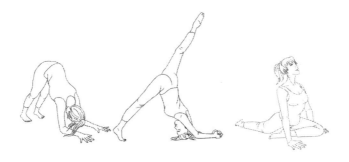

Dolphin Pose - One-Legged Dolphin - Pigeon Pose

PROLAPSED UTERUS

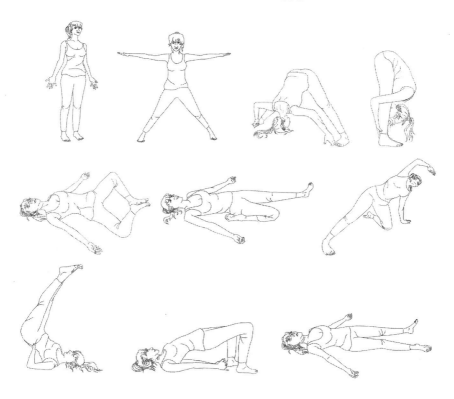

Mountain Pose - Five-Pointed Star - Wide-Legged Forward Bend - Standing Forward Fold - Supine Bound Angle - Half-Supine Hero - Half-Circle - Half Shoulder-Stand - Bridge Pose - Corpse Pose

RESPIRATORY AILMENTS

While doing this sequence, pay special attention to opening your chest. Practice this routine, as well as the one for asthma and colds, to increase the strength of your respiratory system.

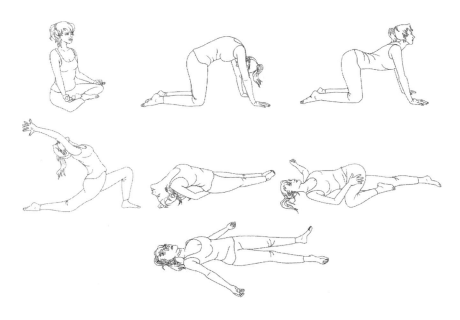

Accomplished Pose (with alternating nostril breathing) - Cat Tilt - Dog Tilt - Low Warrior - Fish Pose - Knee-Down Twist - Corpse Pose

RUNNER'S ACHES AND SHIN SPLINTS

Runner's Aches

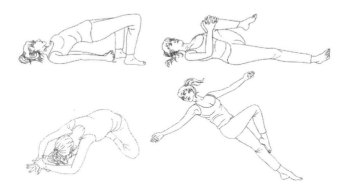

Bridge Pose - Half Wind-Relieving Pose - Seated Head to Knee - Knee-Down Twist

Shin Splints

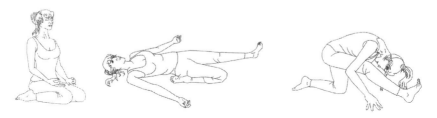

Hero Pose - Half-Supine Hero - Half-Pyramid Pose

SCIATICA

Sciatica Sequence One

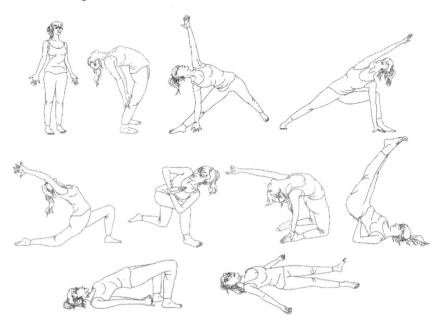

*Mountain Pose - Standing Backbend - Triangle Pose - Extended Side Angle -
Low Warrior - Half Prayer-Twist - Half-Camel - Half Shoulder-Stand -
Bridge Pose - Corpse Pose*

Sciatica Sequence Two

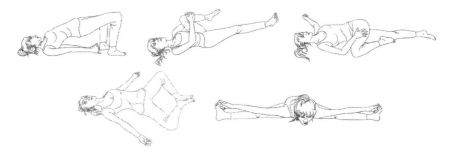

Bridge Pose - Half Wind-Relieving Pose - Knee-Down Twist - Supine Bound Angle - Seated Angle

STOMACH PROBLEMS

Stomach Ache

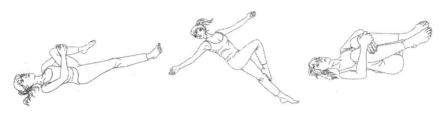

Half Wind-Relieving Pose - Knee-Down Twist - Wind-Relieving Pose

Digestion

This sequence will strengthen your digestive system.

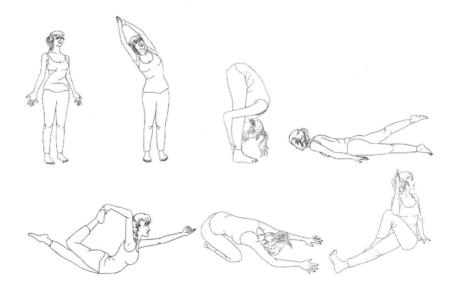

*Mountain Pose - Crescent Moon - Standing Forward Fold - Half Locust -
Half-Bow - Child Pose - Seated Spinal Twist*

Constipation

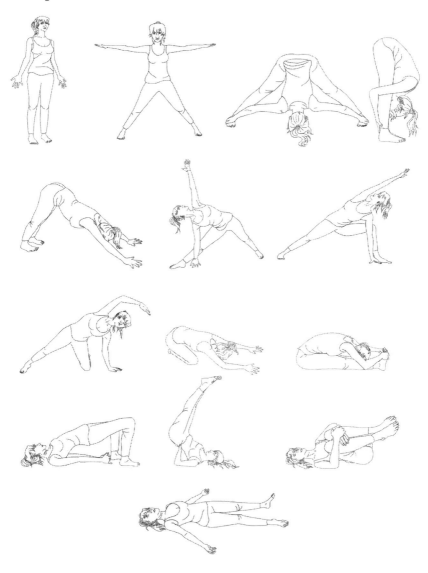

Mountain Pose - Five-Pointed Star - Wide-Legged Forward Bend - Standing Forward Fold - Downward Dog - Triangle Pose - Extended Side Angle - Half-Circle - Child Pose - Seated Forward Bend - Bridge Pose - Half Shoulder-Stand - Wind-Relieving Pose - Corpse Pose

Diarrhea

Ensure that your abdomen is not cramped or restricted while you're doing this sequence.

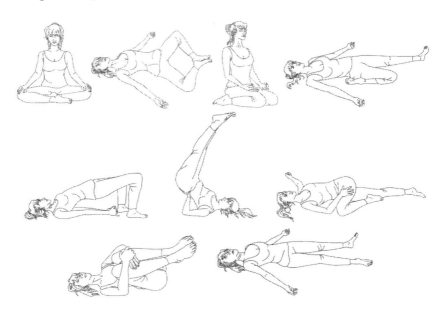

Accomplished Pose - Supine Bound Angle - Hero Pose - Half-Supine Hero - Bridge Pose - Half Shoulder-Stand - Knee-Down Twist - Wind-Relieving Pose - Corpse Pose

STRENGTH

This sequence is good for overall body strength.

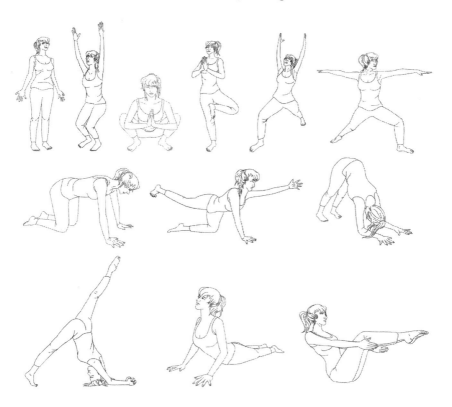

Mountain Pose - Chair Pose - Prayer Squat - Tree Pose - Warrior One - Warrior Two - Table Pose - Balancing Table - Dolphin Pose - One-Legged Dolphin - Cobra Pose - Upward Boat

STRESS AND ANXIETY

Regular practice of these sequences has a long-lasting effect, lowering stress and anxiety. When doing them, keep your whole face relaxed.

Stress and Anxiety Sequence One

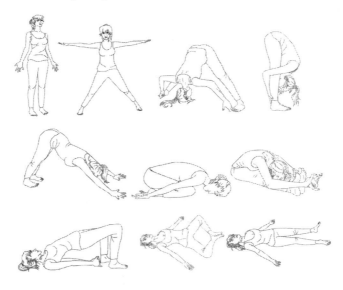

Mountain Pose - Five-Pointed Star - Wide-Legged Forward Bend - Standing Forward Fold - Downward Dog - Child Pose - Seated Forward Bend - Bridge Pose - Supine Bound Angle - Corpse Pose (with Yoga Nidra)

Stress and Anxiety Sequence Two

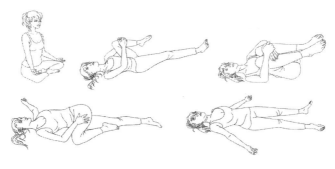

Accomplished Pose (with meditation) - Half Wind-Relieving Pose - Wind-Relieving Pose - Knee-Down Twist - Corpse Pose

Stress and Anxiety Sequence Three

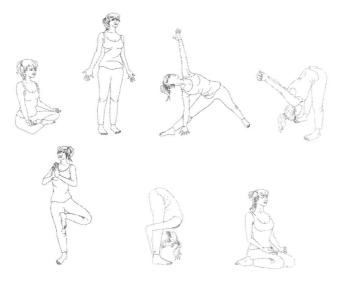

Accomplished Pose (with meditation) - Mountain Pose - Triangle Pose - Standing Yoga Seal - Tree Pose - Standing Forward Fold - Hero Pose (with meditation)

Stress and Anxiety Sequence Four

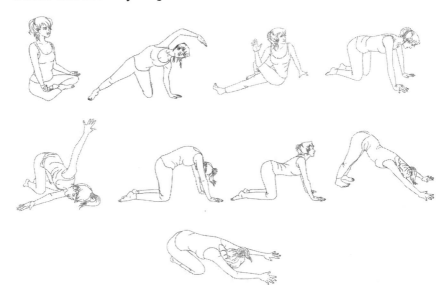

Accomplished Pose (with alternate nostril breathing) - Half-Circle - Seated Spinal Twist - Table Pose - Threading the Needle - Cat Tilt - Dog Tilt - Downward Dog - Child Pose (with meditation)

TENSE SHOULDERS AND NECK

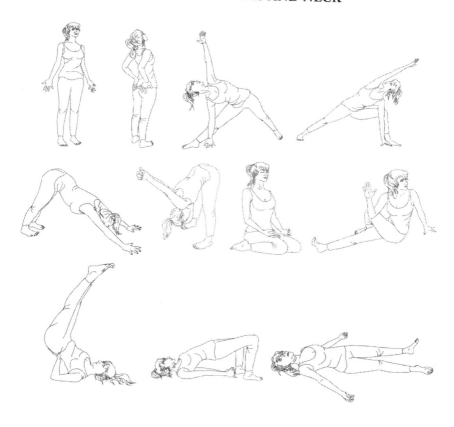

Mountain Pose - Standing Backbend - Triangle Pose - Extended Side Angle -
Downward Dog - Standing Yoga Seal - Hero Pose - Seated Spinal Twist -
Half Shoulder-Stand - Bridge Pose - Corpse Pose

THYROID IMBALANCE

This short routine is aimed at restoring overall balance to the thyroid.

Specific thyroid conditions need specific treatments. Use this sequence as a supplement to your health professional's advised treatment.

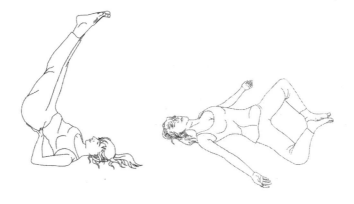

Half Shoulder-Stand - Supine Bound Angle

TOXIN FLUSH

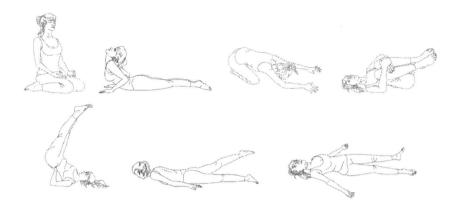

Hero Pose - Cobra Pose - Child Pose - Wind-Relieving Pose - Half Shoulder-Stand - Half Locust - Corpse Pose (with Yoga Nidra)

VARICOSE VEINS

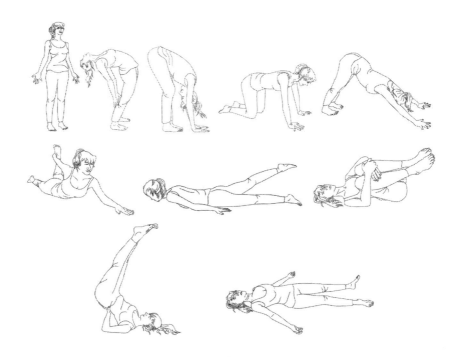

Mountain Pose - Standing Backbend - Standing Forward Fold - Table Pose - Downward Dog - Half-Bow - Half Locust - Wind-Relieving Pose - Half Shoulder-Stand - Corpse Pose

VERTIGO / DIZZY SPELL

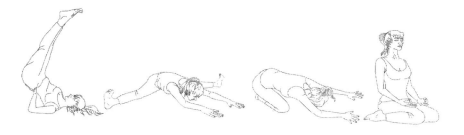

Half Shoulder-Stand - Seated Angle - Child Pose - Hero Pose (with meditation)

Dear Reader,

Thank you for reading *Curing Yoga*.

If you enjoyed it, please leave a review on Amazon. It helps more than most people think. You can do that here:

www.SurvivalFitnessPlan.com/Curing-Yoga-Review-Amazon

Claim your bonus materials:

www.SurvivalFitnessPlan.com/Book-Bonuses

Connect with like-minded people and discuss anything SFP related via the SFP Facebook group:

www.Facebook.com/groups/SurvivalFitnessPlan

A list of resources used in the creation of the Survival Fitness Series is available at:

www.SurvivalFitnessPlan.com/Survival-Fitness-Series

Thanks again for your support,

Aventuras De Viaje.

AUTHOR RECOMMENDATIONS

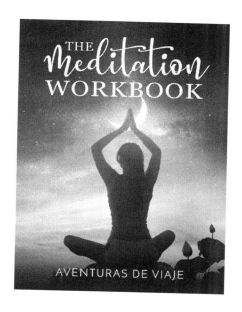

Teach Yourself to Meditate

Discover your inner peace, because this book has 160+ meditations to choose from.

Get it now.

www.SurvivalFitnessPlan.com/Meditation-Workbook

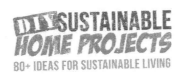

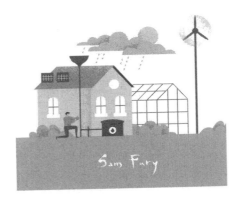

Discover 80+ Sustainable Living Projects

Start making your home more sustainable today, because this book has DIY projects for everyone!

Get it now.

www.SurvivalFitnessPlan.com/DIY-Sustainable-Home-Projects

SURVIVAL FITNESS PLAN TRAINING MANUALS

Survival Fitness

When in danger, you have two options: fight or flight.

This series contains training manuals on the best methods of flight. Together with self-defense, you can train in them for general health and fitness.

- **Parkour.** All the parkour skills you need to overcome obstacles in your path.
- **Climbing.** Focusing on essential bouldering techniques.
- **Riding.** Essential mountain-bike riding techniques. Go as fast as possible in the safest manner.
- **Swimming.** Swimming for endurance and/or speed using the most efficient strokes.

It also has books covering general health and wellness, such as yoga and meditation.

www.SurvivalFitnessPlan.com/Survival-Fitness-Series

Self-Defense

The Self-Defense Series has volumes on some of the martial arts used as a base in SFP self-defense.

It also contains the SFP self-defense training manuals. SFP Self-Defense is an efficient and effective form of minimalist self-defense.

www.SurvivalFitnessPlan.com/Self-Defense-Series

Escape, Evasion, and Survival

SFP escape, evasion, and survival (EES) focuses on keeping you alive using minimal resources. Subjects covered include:

- **Disaster Survival.** How to prepare for and react in the case of disaster and/or societal collapse.
- **Escape and Evasion.** The ability to escape capture and hide from your enemy.
- **Urban and Wilderness Survival.** Being able to live off the land in all terrains.
- **Emergency Roping.** Basic climbing skills and improvised roping techniques.
- **Water Rescue.** Life-saving water skills based on surf life-saving and military training course competencies.
- **Wilderness First Aid.** Modern medicine for use in emergency situations.

www.SurvivalFitnessPlan.com/Escape-Evasion-Survival-Series

Sustainable Living

Create a lifestyle focused on minimal impact to the environment and maximum self-reliance.

SFP sustainable living subjects include permaculture, renewable energy, financial freedom, minimalist living, and more.

www.SurvivalFitnessPlan.com/Sustainable-Living-Series

Miscellaneous

Books by the SFP authors that do not fit into any of the major series.

www.SurvivalFitnessPlan.com/Miscellaneous-Titles

ABOUT THE AUTHOR

Aventuras has three passions: travel, writing, and self-improvement.

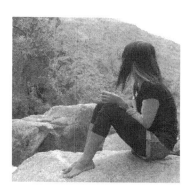

Combining these three things, Miss Viaje spends her time exploring the world and learning about all the things she loves.

She takes what she discovers and shares it through her books.

www.SurvivalFitnessPlan.com

🅰 amazon.com/author/aventuras

🅰 facebook.com/SurvivalFitnessPlan

🅰 twitter.com/Survival_Fitnes

🅰 pinterest.com/survivalfitnes

🅰 goodreads.com/MissAventurasDeViaje

🅰 bookbub.com/authors/aventuras-de-viaje

Printed in Germany
by Amazon Distribution
GmbH, Leipzig